AF889097

Official Journal of the International Society for Neuroimmunomodulation

NeuroImmunoModulation

Founded 1994 by S.M. McCann and J.M. Lipton
Continued by G.P. Chrousos (2002–2006)

KARGER

Printed in Germany on acid-free and non-aging paper
(ISO 9706) by Stückle Druck, Ettenheim

Guidelines for Authors

NeuroImmunoModulation

Aims and Scope

The rapidly expanding area of research known as neuroimmunomodulation explores the way in which the nervous system interacts with the immune system via neural, hormonal, and paracrine actions. Encompassing both basic and clinical research, *Neuroimmunomodulation* reports on all aspects of these interactions. Basic investigations consider all neural and humoral interactions from molecular genetics through cell regulation to integrative systems of the body. The journal also aims to clarify the basic mechanisms involved in the pathogenesis of the CNS pathology in AIDS patients and in various neurodegenerative diseases. Although primarily devoted to research articles, timely reviews will be published on a regular basis. To ensure high quality, all papers will be reviewed by at least two referees, with every effort made to maintain a short publication time.

Manuscripts

should be submitted using the online submission website at:

www.karger.com/nim

Authors are asked to suggest three to four potential reviewers for their manuscript. These experts on the topic of the article should not be from the same institution as the author(s). The names and the full postal and e-mail addresses of potential reviewers should be submitted with each article. Editors will consider these suggestions but are not bound by them.

Should you experience any problems with your submission, please contact the Editorial Office:

nim@karger.com

Conditions

All manuscripts are subject to editorial review. Manuscripts are received with the explicit understanding that they are not under simultaneous consideration by any other publication. Submission of an article for publication implies the transfer of the copyright from the author to the publisher upon acceptance. Accepted papers become the permanent property of *Neuroimmunomodulation* and may not be reproduced by any means, in whole or in part, without the written consent of the publisher. It is the author's responsibility to obtain permission to reproduce illustrations, tables, etc. from other publications.

Most reviews are solicited by the editors. Unsolicited reviews may also be considered, but authors should send a brief proposal to the editorial office, summarizing the topic of the proposed review and 4–5 key references.

Manuscripts should be written in English. They should contain unpublished results of research work, and should be as concise as possible. They should be typewritten on 'letter-quality' paper printed on one side of the sheet only and double spaced with a wide margin. Please send the original and three first-class copies of the manuscript. One set of the original illustrations plus three copies is adequate, except in the case of photomicrographs or other illustrations that do not reproduce well in Xerox or related types of copying equipment. In these instances, it will be necessary to submit four clear prints of each illustration for distribution to the reviewers. The final version of your manuscript and illustrations should be submitted on disk. For details refer to 'Disk Submission' or www.karger.com/journals/disksub.htm. Editorial review and copyediting will be executed from the disk version of your manuscript. The following presentation is recommended: Abstract, Introductory statement on the purpose of the studies, Materials and Methods, Results, Discussion, and References. Commonly accepted abbreviations (e.g. ACTH, TSH, DNA) may be used throughout the text and tables, but a definition should be provided the first time each abbreviation is used. Please limit abbreviations to those in common use, and avoid other abbreviations and acronyms. Contributions will generally be printed in order of acceptance for publication. Contributors should know that one of the criteria considered in reviewing manuscripts is the humane and proper treatment of animals. The editors realize that the use of anesthetics, analgesics, and tranquilizers would defeat the purpose of some experiments. However, the use of painful or otherwise noxious stimuli must be carefully and thoroughly justified in the paper. Papers that do not meet these criteria will not be accepted for publication.

Rapid communications: Manuscripts intended for rapid communication must present new findings of sufficient importance to justify their accelerated appearance. Double-spaced manuscripts cannot exceed 7 pages, including figures, tables and references; longer manuscripts will be returned. Rapid communications are subject to the usual editorial review and are published within 2 months following acceptance. Proofs are sent to the Editors and to the authors.

Arrangement

All pages should be numbered consecutively and carry the author's name in the upper right corner.

Title page: The first page of each paper should carry the title, the authors' full first and last names, and the name of the institute or department where the authors conducted their research work. In addition, the following should be put on the title page: 1. A short title for use as a running head; 2. A list of 3–9 key words that reflect the content of the paper; 3. The name and complete mailing address, phone and fax numbers as well as e-mail address of the individual to whom correspondence, proofs, and requests for reprints should be addressed.

***Abstract:* Each paper needs an abstract of up to 250 words. Abstracts for Original Papers should be structured with subheadings as follows: Objective(s), Methods, Results, Conclusion(s). The words used in the subheadings of the Abstract are not included in the 250 words of the Abstract.**

Footnotes: Avoid footnotes if at all possible. When essential, they should be numbered consecutively and typed at the foot of the appropriate page.

Tables and illustrations: Tables (numbered in arabic numerals) should be prepared on separate sheets, and each should have a suitable heading. Illustrations should be numbered in Arabic numerals and legends for the figures should be submitted on a separate page. For the reproduction of illustrations, only good drawings and original photographs can be accepted; negatives or photocopies cannot be used. Due to technical reasons, figures with a screen background should not be submitted. When possible, group several illustrations on one block for reproduction (max. size 180 × 223 mm) or provide crop marks. On the back of each illustration, indicate its number, the author's name, and 'top' with a soft pencil. Electronically submitted b/w half-tone and color illustrations must have a final resolution of 300 dpi after scaling, line drawings one of 800–1,200 dpi.

Color illustrations

Online edition: Color illustrations are reproduced free of charge. In the print version, the illustrations are reproduced in black and white. Please avoid referring to the colors in the text and figure legends.

Print edition: Up to 6 color illustrations per page can be integrated within the text at CHF 800.00 per page.

Acknowledgments, including, where relevant, credit to the sources of grant support, should be placed before the references.

References: In the text identify references by Arabic numerals [in square brackets]. Material submitted for publication but not yet accepted should be noted as [unpublished data] and not be included in the reference list. The list of references should include only those publications which are cited in the text. Do not alphabetize; number references in the order in which they are first mentioned in the text. The surnames of all the authors followed by initials should be given. There should be no punctuation other than a comma to separate the authors. Preferably, please cite all authors. Abbreviate journal names according to the Index Medicus system. Also see International Committee of Medical Journal Editors: Uniform requirements for manuscripts submitted to biomedical journals (www.icmje.org).

Examples

(a) Papers published in periodicals: Sun J, Koto H, Chung KF: Interaction of ozone and allergen challenges on bronchial responsiveness and inflammation in sensitised guinea pigs. Int Arch Allergy Immunol 1997;112:191–195.

(b) Papers published only with DOI numbers:
Theoharides TC, Boucher W, Spear K: Serum interleukin-6 reflects disease severity and osteoporosis in mastocytosis patients. Int Arch Allergy Immunol DOI: 10.1159/000063858.

(c) Monographs: Matthews DE, Farewell VT: Using and Understanding Medical Statistics, ed 3, revised. Basel, Karger, 1996.

(d) Edited books: Parren PWHI, Burton DR: Antibodies against HIV-1 from phage display libraries: Mapping of an immune response and progress towards antiviral immunotherapy; in Capra JD (ed): Antibody Engineering. Chem Immunol. Basel, Karger, 1997, vol 65, pp 18–56.

(e) Papers published in electronic format: Black CA: Delayed type hypersensitivity: Current theories with a historic perspective. Dermatol Online J 1999;5:7. http://dermatology.cdlib.org/DOJvol5num1.

Papers that have been submitted to a journal but are not yet accepted should not be listed in the bibliography, but the data in them can be referred to in the text as unpublished observations. If details of methods are only available in papers that are 'in press', copies of the papers should be included with the manuscript submitted to *Neuroimmunomodulation*, so that the editorial referees can have adequate information to judge the manuscript.

Reference Management Software: Use of EndNote is recommended for easy management and formatting of citations and reference lists.

Digital Object Identifier (DOI)

S. Karger Publishers supports DOIs as unique identifiers for articles. A DOI number will be printed on the title page of each article. DOIs can be useful in the future for identifying and citing articles published online without volume or issue information. More information can be found at www.doi.org.

Supplementary Material

Supplementary material is restricted to additional data that are not necessary for the scientific integrity and conclusions of the paper. Please note that all supplementary files will undergo editorial review and should be submitted together with the original manuscript. The Editors reserve the right to limit the scope and length of the supplementary material. Supplementary material must meet production quality standards for Web publication without the need for any modification or editing. In general, supplementary files should not exceed 10 Mb in size. All figures and tables should have titles and legends and all files should be supplied separately and named clearly. Acceptable files and formats are: Word or PDF files, Excel spreadsheets (only if the data cannot be converted properly to a PDF file), and video files (.mov, .avi, .mpeg).

Author's Choice™

Karger's Author's Choice™ service broadens the reach of your article and gives all users worldwide free and full access for reading, downloading and printing at www.karger.com. The option is available for a one-time fee of CHF 3,000.00, which is a permissible cost in grant allocation. More information can be found at www.karger.com/authors_choice.

NIH-Funded Research

The U.S. National Institutes of Health (NIH) mandates under the NIH Public Access Policy that final, peer-reviewed manuscripts appear in its digital database within 12 months of the official publication date. As a service to authors, Karger submits the final version of your article on your behalf to PubMed Central. For those selecting our premium Author's Choice™ service, we will send your article immediately upon publishing, accelerating the accessibility of your work without the usual embargo. More details on NIH's Public Access Policy is available at http://publicaccess.nih.gov/policy.htm

Self-Archiving

Karger permits authors to archive their pre-prints (i.e. pre-refereeing) or post-prints (i.e. final draft post-refereeing) on their personal or institution's servers, provided the following conditions are met: Articles may not be used for commercial purposes, must be linked to the publisher's version, and must acknowledge the publisher's copyright. Authors selecting Karger's Author's Choice™ feature, however, are also permitted to archive the final, published version of their article, which includes copyediting and design improvements as well as citation links.

Electronic Proofs

Unless indicated otherwise, proofs will be e-mailed to the corresponding author.

Reprints

Order forms and a price list are sent with the proofs. Orders submitted after the issue is printed are subject to considerably higher prices.

KARGER

E-Mail karger@karger.com
www.karger.com

The Guidelines for Authors are available at:
www.karger.com/nim_Guidelines

General Information

NeuroImmunoModulation

ISSN Print Edition: 1021–7401
ISSN Online Edition: 1423–0216

Journal Homepage: www.karger.com/nim

Publication Data: *Neuroimmunomodulation* is published 6 times a year. Volume 22 with 6 issues appears in 2015.

Subscription Rates: Subscriptions run for a full calendar year. Prices are given per year.

Personal subscription:

Print or Online	Print+Online combined
CHF 697.00	CHF 745.00
EUR 580.00	EUR 619.00
USD 711.00	USD 759.00

postage and handling (added to print and print+online)
CHF 45.60 Europe, CHF 67.20 Overseas
EUR 38.40
USD 62.40

Institutional subscription:

Print or Online	Print+Online combined
CHF 1990.00	CHF 2289.00
EUR 1658.00	EUR 1907.00
USD 20310.00	USD 2336.00

postage and handling (added to print and print+online)
CHF 57.00 Europe, CHF 84.00 Overseas
EUR 48.00
USD 78.00

Please enquire about reduced rates for members of the: International Society of Neuroimmunomodulation

Back Volumes and Single Issues: Information on availability and prices of single print issues and print or electronic back volumes can be obtained from Customer Service at *service@karger.com.*

Bibliographic Indices: This journal is regularly listed in bibliographic services, including *Current Contents*® and PubMed/MEDLINE.

Subscription Orders:
Orders can be placed at agencies, bookstores, directly with the Publisher

S. Karger AG
Medical and Scientific Publishers
Allschwilerstrasse 10
CH–4009 Basel
Switzerland

t: +41 61 306 11 11
f: +41 61 306 12 34
e: karger@karger.com
w: www.karger.com

(for courier services only:
Allschwilerstrasse 10
CH–4055 Basel)

or further Karger offices or representatives:

Germany
S. Karger GmbH
Postfach
79095 Freiburg
Deutschland
(Hausadresse: Wilhelmstrasse 20A, 79098 Freiburg)
t: +49 761 45 20 70
f: +49 761 45 20 714
e: information@karger.de
w: www.karger.de

Japan
Karger Japan, Inc.
Shiba Daimon Asahi Bldg. 2F
1-2-23 Shiba Daimon
Minato-ku
Tokyo 105-0012
Japan
t: +81 3 6435 6242
f: +81 3 6435 6244
e: publisher@karger.jp
w: www.karger.jp

USA
S. Karger Publishers, Inc.
26 West Avon Road
P.O. Box 529
Unionville, CT 06085
USA
Toll free: +1 800 828 5479
t: +1 860 675 7834
f: +1 860 675 7302
e: karger@snet.net

France
Enter & Read
Albertine Luginbuhl
23, rue du Départ, boite 37
75014 Paris
France
t: +33 (0) 6 81 04 76 85
e: albertineluginbuhl@orange.fr

South East Asia, China and Taiwan
Karger Regional Office (Malaysia)
Level 28-03-03A, PJ Exchange
No. 16A, Persiaran Barat
46050 Petaling Jaya
Selangor Darul Ehsan
Malaysia
t: +60 3 7962 0158
f: +60 3 7962 0001
e: service@karger.cn; r.chew@karger.cn

Karger China
West/5F, China Life Tower
No.16, Chao Wai Street
Chaoyang District
Beijing 100020
China
t: +86 10 5877 1408
f: +86 10 5877 1120
e: service@karger.cn; r.chew@karger.cn
w: www.karger.cn

India, Bangladesh, Sri Lanka
Karger India
Plot No. 17, Yusuf Sarai Market
B.L. Glass Building, 2nd Floor
Sri Aurobindo Marg
New Delhi 110 016
India
t: +91 11 46029 633
f: +91 11 46029 634
c: +91 98 91052 128
e: r.kumar@kargerindia.com
w: www.karger.com

Change of Address:
Both old and new address should be sent to the subscription source.

KARGER

E-Mail karger@karger.com
www.karger.com

The Journal Home Page is available at:
www.karger.com/nim

Providing an overview of the most recent advances and breakthrough developments

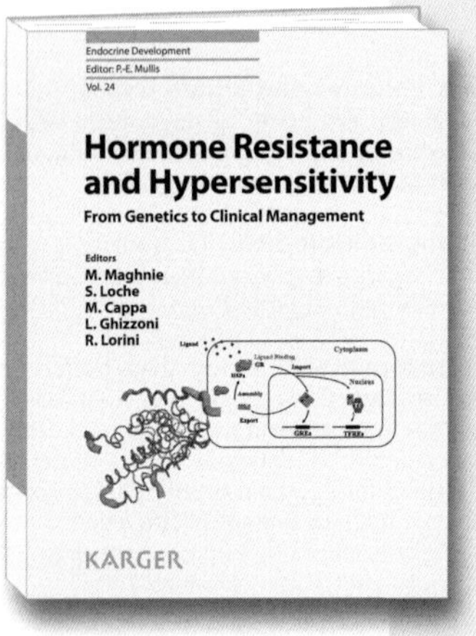

Hormone Resistance and Hypersensitivity

From Genetics to Clinical Management

Editors
Mohamad Maghnie
Sandro Loche
Marco Cappa
Lucia Ghizzoni
Renata Lorini

Hormone Resistance and Hypersensitivity
From Genetics to Clinical Management
Editors: Maghnie, M. (Genoa);
Loche, S. (Cagliari); Cappa, M. (Rome);
Ghizzoni, L. (Turin); Lorini, R. (Genoa)
VIII + 160 p., 26 fig., 7 in color, 10 tab., 2013
CHF 168.– / EUR 140.– / USD 198.00 (hard cover)
CHF 202.– / EUR 168.– / USD 238.00 (online)
Online version for institutional purchase
Prices subject to change
EUR price for Germany, USD price for USA only
ISBN 978–3–318–02267–4 (hard cover)
e-ISBN 978–3–318–02268–1

Endocrine Development, Vol. 24
Series Editor: P.-E. Mullis (Bern)

Over recent years, impressive advances in genetic/epigenetic technology have greatly improved the understanding of the pathogenesis of pediatric endocrine diseases due to hormone resistance and hypersensitivity.
This book presents reviews of thyroid hormone and thyroid hormone receptor resistance, and genetics and epigenetics of parathyroid hormone resistance. Abnormalities of the pituitary-gonadal axis affecting puberty as well as androgen receptor are covered. Novel insights into the diseases affecting ACTH, glucocorticoid and aldosterone receptors are discussed. Further chapters address new aspects of the physiology of the GH and IGF-1 axis as well as the diseases related to GH-IGF-1 receptor and post-receptor signaling defects. A key chapter on metabolic insights into insulin resistance is also included.
Covering clinical and genetic aspects of hormone resistance and hypersensitivity, this book will be a useful tool in the hands of scientists, physicians and other healthcare professionals who wish to be up to date with novel research findings in this area.

Contents

Dear Librarian

I have reviewed this publication and would like to recommend it for our library.

Recommended by: ____________________

Department: ____________________

Date: ____________________

Signature: ____________________

Orders may be placed with any bookshop, subscription agency, directly with the publisher or through a Karger distributor.

The easiest way to order: **www.karger.com/endev**

Karger – Medical and Scientific Publishers
CH–4009 Basel, Switzerland
orders@karger.com, f: +41 61 306 12 34
www.karger.com

KI 13622

KARGER

NeuroImmunoModulation

Low-Dose Glucocorticoids in Rheumatic Diseases

Editors
Maurizio Cutolo, Genoa
George P. Chrousos, Athens
Theodore Pincus, Chicago, Ill.

27 figures and 16 tables, 2015

KARGER
Basel · Freiburg · Paris · London · New York · Chennai · New Delhi · Bangkok · Beijing · Shanghai · Tokyo · Kuala Lumpur · Singapore · Sydney

S. Karger
Medical and Scientific Publishers
Basel · Freiburg · Paris · London ·
New York · Chennai · New Delhi ·
Bangkok · Beijing · Shanghai · Tokyo ·
Kuala Lumpur · Singapore · Sydney

Disclaimer
The statements, opinions and data contained in this publication are solely those of the individual authors and contributors and not of the publisher and the editor(s). The appearance of advertisements in the journal is not a warranty, endorsement, or approval of the products or services advertised or of their effectiveness, quality or safety. The publisher and the editor(s) disclaim responsibility for any injury to persons or property resulting from any ideas, methods, instructions or products referred to in the content or advertisements.

Drug Dosage
The authors and the publisher have exerted every effort to ensure that drug selection and dosage set forth in this text are in accord with current recommendations and practice at the time of publication. However, in view of ongoing research, changes in government regulations, and the constant flow of information relating to drug therapy and drug reactions, the reader is urged to check the package insert for each drug for any change in indications and dosage and for added warnings and precautions. This is particularly important when the recommended agent is a new and/or infrequently employed drug.

P.O. Box, CH–4009 Basel (Switzerland)
Printed in Germany
on acid-free and non-aging paper (ISO 9706) by
Stückle Druck, Ettenheim
ISBN 978–3–318–02711–2
e-ISBN 978–3–318–02712–9

KARGER

E-Mail karger@karger.com
www.karger.com/nim

NeuroImmunoModulation

Neuroimmunomodulation 2015;22:3–5
DOI: 10.1159/000362737

Published online: September 12, 2014

Special Issue on Glucocorticoid Therapy in Rheumatic Diseases: Introduction

The co-editors, Maurizio Cutolo, George P. Chrousos and Theodore Pincus, are pleased to present this special issue of *Neuroimmunology,* concerning contemporary use of low-dose glucocorticoids in the treatment of patients with rheumatic diseases. Prednisolone was introduced for the treatment of rheumatoid arthritis (RA) in 1949 [1]. Spectacular results were documented not only in the medical literature, but also in a short film and descriptions in US national magazines. The 1950 Nobel Prize in Medicine and Physiology was awarded to Hench and collaborators for their achievement [2].

In 1949, the time of the discovery of the clinical benefits of prednisolone, new medications could be introduced for marketing without evidence of superiority to placebo in randomized controlled clinical trials, which was introduced only in the 1940s [3, 4]. Furthermore, no requirement existed to analyze the risk/benefit ratio or dose-response relations at different doses. Therefore, guidelines were not available concerning optimal dosages for different indications, or for how long therapy should be continued.

In 1955, the Mayo Clinic group that discovered the use of clinical prednisone actually suggested that doses of <7.5 mg of prednisolone per day appeared clinically efficacious for RA [5]. However, it was widely believed that such low doses could not slow radiographic progression and be disease modifying [6]. For example, the Empire Rheumatism Council Studies, which documented in 1957 that glucocorticoids slowed radiographic progression [7], involved initial doses of 75 mg per day of cortisone acetate, equivalent to 15 mg per day of prednisolone (18.75 mg per day of prednisone).

In the 1950s, glucocorticoids were by far the most potent available anti-inflammatory therapy, usually administered as monotherapy to patients with RA and other rheumatic diseases. As monotherapy, rheumatic diseases were treated with doses that were often far higher than doses used today, such as 15–60 mg of prednisone per day for RA patients, initially and over lengthy periods [8]. These doses often led to substantial adverse events in most patients within a few months, and might not be recommended at this time when the standard of patient care involves combinations of glucocorticoids with other anti-inflammatory, immunosuppressive, cytotoxic and/or biologic agents, rather than a monotherapy.

By the late 1950s, glucocorticoids were recommended for RA primarily as intra-articular and intramuscular therapy [8]. Oral glucocorticoids were regarded primarily as a 'bridging therapy', until disease-modifying antirheumatic drugs would become efficacious, or for patients with life-threatening vasculitis or other severe extra-articular disease. RA was not regarded as a 'fatal' disease, and discontinuation of oral glucocorticoids within a few months has been recommended for decades. Even the 2014 EULAR guidelines for management of RA suggest that oral glucocorticoids be continued for 6

KARGER

1021–7401/14/0222–0003$39.50/0

E-Mail karger@karger.com
www.karger.com/nim

months [9]. Long -term glucocorticoids, even at low doses, remain regarded as undesirable and strongly contraindicated.

Despite admonitions in textbooks and the rheumatology literature, glucocorticoids remain a mainstay for treatment of RA and other inflammatory rheumatic diseases. For example, in the international QUEST-RA study reported in 2008, 71% of all 6,004 RA patients studied had taken prednisone at some time – more than 50% of patients in 23 of 26 countries, the 3 exceptions being Denmark (44%), the Netherlands (41%) and Russia (44%) [10]. Many of these patients are treated over long periods, as withdrawal of prednisone as recommended is associated with a resurgence of symptoms in many patients who are more comfortable maintaining low doses of prednisone. In SLE, among 539 patients monitored in the Johns Hopkins Lupus Cohort, 89% had been treated with glucocorticoids, and 57% of patients with a disease duration >10 years had always received these agents [11]. Almost all patients with vasculitis, polymyositis, polymyalgia rheumatica and most other inflammatory rheumatic diseases are treated with glucocorticoids.

Historically, it is of interest that one clinical trial was reported by de Andrade et al. [6] in 1964, which compared treatment with 5 mg of prednisone per day in the morning versus 5 mg per day in the evening. The authors reported that the evening dose was preferred by the majority of patients. They also noted that many patients in their clinical setting had never taken a dose greater than 7.5 mg per day (on the basis of recommendations from the Mayo Clinic group [5]), and most never more than 5 mg per day [6]. However, this practice did not become widespread, possibly in part because even these investigators and the rheumatology community did not believe 5 mg could be disease modifying in RA [6] (see article by Pincus et al., this issue p. 46).

A reassessment of oral glucocorticoids for treatment of RA began in the mid-1980s, concomitant with recognition that the long-term consequences of RA were more severe than had been recognized previously, including frequent work disability [12, 13], early radiographic damage within the first 2 years of disease [14], and premature mortality rates [13, 15, 16]. Mortality rates in patients with severe RA were similar to those seen in severe hypertension and diabetes [17]. These observations modified concepts concerning the risk/benefit ratio of glucocorticoids for RA. (Even at present, patients with neoplastic disease may be treated with doses of prednisone of 60 mg per day for months, without any recommendations that these doses may have a long-term negative risk/benefit ratio.)

A non-blinded clinical trial of 5 mg of prednisone per day was reported by Harris et al. [18] in 1983 to result in both improved functional capacity and slowing of radiographic progression compared to placebo. In the 1990s, Kirwan [19] and Boers et al. [20] conducted influential clinical trials documenting both disease modification and clinical improvement with doses of 7.5 mg of prednisolone. In the 2000s, six additional clinical trials documented disease modification with prednisolone of 10 mg per day or less [21–26], including one trial with 5 mg per day [23]. A withdrawal clinical trial documented that patients could detect differences between placebo and 3 mg of prednisone [24]; even 3 mg of prednisone appears to be disease modifying, as these patients had only 3% of maximum radiographic scores over 8 years or longer [27]. Recently, modified-release prednisone was introduced to provide greater optimization of prednisone therapy, to be taken at 10 p.m. with release of prednisone at 2 a.m., with documentation of decreased morning stiffness and IL-6 levels compared to standard morning doses [28, 29].

Doses of 5 mg per day or less do not affect the hypothalamic-pituitary-adrenal axis [30–33], as is seen with doses of 10 mg or more. The primary adverse effects seen with doses of 5 mg or less involve skin thinning and bruising; many patients are not affected, and many who are generally accept this problem for the well-being they gain from low-dose glucocorticoids [6, 27]. By contrast, long-term doses of 10 mg or more are associated with increased cardiovascular disease and other adverse events [34]. Therefore, low doses of prednisone may be as beneficial as high doses are harmful [35].

This special issue includes four categories of articles under the headings: (1) basic research concerning glucocorticoids; (2) efficacy of low-dose glucocorticoids in clinical trials; (3) safety of low-dose glucocorticoids in rheumatoid arthritis, and (4) observational studies and clinical experience with low-dose glucocorticoids. We thank the authors for their excellent contributions, and hope that readers will find them interesting and informative. We hope that this special issue will contribute to scientific knowledge concerning optimal clinical use of glucocorticoids, toward improved outcomes of patients with RA and all inflammatory rheumatic diseases. The authors and co-editors welcome comments from readers.

Maurizio Cutolo, Genoa
George P. Chrousos, Athens
Theodore Pincus, Chicago, Ill.

References

1 Hench PS, Kendall EC, Slocumb CH, Polley HF: The effect of a hormone of the adrenal cortex (17-hydroxy-11-dehydrocorticosterone; compound E) and of the pituitary adrenocorticotropic hormone on rheumatoid arthritis. Proc Staff Meet Mayo Clin 1949;24:181–197.

2 Hench PS: The reversibility of certain rheumatic and non-rheumatic conditions by the use of cortisone or of the pituitary adrenocorticotropic hormone. Ann Intern Med 1952;36:1–38.

3 Medical Resarch Council: Streptomycin treatment of pulmonary tuberculosis. Br Med J 1948;2:769–782.

4 Hill AB: Suspended judgment: memories of the British streptomycin trial in tuberculosis – the first randomized clinical trial. Controlled Clin Trials 1990;11:77–79.

5 Polley HF, Slocumb CH, Ward LE, Hench PS: Recognition and treatment of patients with chronic hypercortisonism. Ann Rheum Dis 1955;14(4):416–417.

6 de Andrade JR, McCormick JN, Hill AGS: Small doses of prednisolone in the management of rheumatoid arthritis. Ann Rheum Dis 1964;23:158–162.

7 Empire Rheumatism Council: Multi-centre controlled trial comparing cortisone acetate and acetyl salicylic acid in the long-term treatment of rheumatoid arthritis: results of three years treatment. Ann Rheum Dis 1957;16:277–289.

8 West HF: Rheumatoid arthritis: the relevance of clinical knowledge to research activities. Abstr World Med 1967;41:401–417.

9 Smolen JS, Landewe R, Breedveld FC, Buch M, Burmester G, Dougados M, et al: EULAR recommendations for the management of rheumatoid arthritis with synthetic and biological disease-modifying antirheumatic drugs: 2013 update. Ann Rheum Dis 2014;73:492–509.

10 Sokka T, Kautiainen H, Pincus T, Toloza S, da Rocha Castelar Pinheiro G, Lazovskis J, et al: Disparities in rheumatoid arthritis disease activity according to gross domestic product in 25 countries in the QUEST-RA database. Ann Rheum Dis 2009;68:1666–1672.

11 Zonana-Nacach A, Barr SG, Magder LS, Petri M: Damage in systemic lupus erythematosus and its association with corticosteroids. Arthritis Rheum 2000;43:1801–1808.

12 Yelin E, Meenan R, Nevitt M, Epstein W: Work disability in rheumatoid arthritis: effects of disease, social, and work factors. Ann Intern Med 1980;93:551–556.

13 Pincus T, Callahan LF, Sale WG, Brooks AL, Payne LE, Vaughn WK: Severe functional declines, work disability, and increased mortality in seventy-five rheumatoid arthritis patients studied over nine years. Arthritis Rheum 1984;27:864–872.

14 Scott DL, Grindulis KA, Struthers GR, Coulton BL, Popert AJ, Bacon PA: Progression of radiological changes in rheumatoid arthritis. Ann Rheum Dis 1984;43:8–17.

15 Isomäki HA, Mutru O, Koota K: Death rate and causes of death in patients with rheumatoid arthritis. Scand J Rheumatol 1975;4:205–208.

16 Rasker JJ, Cosh JA: The natural history of rheumatoid arthritis: a fifteen year follow-up study: the prognostic significance of features noted in the first year. Clin Rheumatol 1984;3:11–20.

17 Pincus T, Callahan LF, Vaughn WK: Questionnaire, walking time and button test measures of functional capacity as predictive markers for mortality in rheumatoid arthritis. J Rheumatol 1987;14:240–251.

18 Harris ED Jr, Emkey RD, Nichols JE, Newberg A: Low dose prednisone therapy in rheumatoid arthritis: a double blind study. J Rheumatol 1983;10:713–721.

19 Kirwan JR: The effects of glucocorticoids on joint destruction in rheumatoid arthritis. N Engl J Med 1995;333:142–146.

20 Boers M, Verhoeven AC, Markusse HM, van de Laar MAFJ, Westhovens R, van Denderen JC, et al: Randomised comparison of combined step-down prednisolone, methotrexate and sulphasalazine with sulphasalazine alone in early rheumatoid arthritis. Lancet 1997;350:309–318.

21 van Everdingen AA, Jacobs JWG, van Reesema DRS, Bijlsma JWJ: Low-dose prednisone therapy for patients with early active rheumatoid arthritis: clinical efficacy, disease-modifying properties, and side effects. Ann Intern Med 2002;136:1–12.

22 Svensson B, Boonen A, Albertsson K, van der Heijde D, Keller C, Hafstrom I: Low-dose prednisolone in addition to the initial disease-modifying antirheumatic drug in patients with early active rheumatoid arthritis reduces joint destruction and increases the remission rate: a two-year randomized trial. Arthritis Rheum 2005;52:3360–3370.

23 Wassenberg S, Rau R, Steinfeld P, Zeidler H: Very low-dose prednisolone in early rheumatoid arthritis retards radiographic progression over two years: a multicenter, double-blind, placebo-controlled trial. Arthritis Rheum 2005;52:3371–3380.

24 Pincus T, Swearingen CJ, Luta G, Sokka T: Efficacy of prednisone 1–4 mg/day in patients with rheumatoid arthritis: a randomised, double-blind, placebo controlled withdrawal clinical trial. Ann Rheum Dis 2009;68:1715–1720.

25 Bakker MF, Jacobs JW, Welsing PM, Verstappen SM, Tekstra J, Ton E, et al: Low-dose prednisone inclusion in a methotrexate-based, tight control strategy for early rheumatoid arthritis: a randomized trial. Ann Intern Med 2012;156:329–339.

26 Montecucco C, Todoerti M, Sakellariou G, Scire CA, Caporali R: Low-dose oral prednisone improves clinical and ultrasonographic remission rates in early rheumatoid arthritis: results of a 12-month open-label randomised study. Arthritis Res Ther 2012;14:R112.

27 Pincus T, Sokka T, Castrejón I, Cutolo M: Decline of mean initial prednisone dosage from 10.3 to 3.6 mg/day to treat rheumatoid arthritis between 1980 and 2004 in one clinical setting, with long-term effectiveness of dosages less than 5 mg/day. Arthritis Care Res 2013;65:729–736.

28 Buttgereit F, Doering G, Schaeffler A, Witte S, Sierakowski S, Gromnica-Ihle E, et al: Efficacy of modified-release versus standard prednisone to reduce duration of morning stiffness of the joints in rheumatoid arthritis (CAPRA-1): a double-blind, randomised controlled trial. Lancet 2008;371:205–214.

29 Buttgereit F, Mehta D, Kirwan J, Szechinski J, Boers M, Alten RE, et al: Low-dose prednisone chronotherapy for rheumatoid arthritis: a randomised clinical trial (CAPRA-2). Ann Rheum Dis 2013;72:204–210.

30 Danowski TS, Bonessi JV, Sabeh G, Sutton RD, Webster MW Jr, Sarver ME: Probabilities of pituitary-adrenal responsiveness after steroid therapy. Ann Intern Med 1964;61:11–26.

31 Wood JB, Frankland AW, James VH, Landon J: A rapid test of adrenocortical function. Lancet 1965;1:243–245.

32 Daly JR, Myles AB, Bacon PA, Beardwell CG, Savage O: Pituitary adrenal function during corticosteroid withdrawal in rheumatoid arthritis. Ann Rheum Dis 1967;26:18–25.

33 LaRochelle GE Jr, LaRochelle AG, Ratner RE, Borenstein DG: Recovery of the hypothalamic-pituitary-adrenal (HPA) axis in patients with rheumatic diseases receiving low-dose prednisone. Am J Med 1993;95:258–264.

34 Wei L, MacDonald TM, Walker BR: Taking glucocorticoids by prescription is associated with subsequent cardiovascular disease. Ann Intern Med 2004;141:764–770.

35 Pincus T, Sokka T, Stein CM: Are long-term very low doses of prednisone for patients with rheumatoid arthritis as helpful as high doses are harmful? Ann Intern Med 2002;136:76–78.

Basic Research concerning Glucocorticoids

NeuroImmunoModulation

Neuroimmunomodulation 2015;22:6–19
DOI: 10.1159/000362736

Published online: September 12, 2014

Stress, the Stress System and the Role of Glucocorticoids

Nicolas C. Nicolaides[a, b] Elli Kyratzi[b] Agaristi Lamprokostopoulou[b]
George P. Chrousos[a–c] Evangelia Charmandari[a, b]

[a]Division of Endocrinology, Metabolism and Diabetes, First Department of Pediatrics, University of Athens Medical School, 'Aghia Sophia' Children's Hospital, and [b]Division of Endocrinology and Metabolism, Clinical Research Center, Biomedical Research Foundation of the Academy of Athens, Athens, Greece; [c]Saudi Diabetes Study Research Group, King Fahd Medical Research Center, King Abdulaziz University, Jeddah, Saudi Arabia

Key Words

Stress system · Stress response · Glucocorticoids · Glucocorticoid receptor · Hypothalamic-pituitary-adrenal axis

Abstract

All living organisms have developed a highly conserved and regulatory system, the stress system, to cope with a broad spectrum of stressful stimuli that threaten, or are perceived as threatening, their dynamic equilibrium or homeostasis. This neuroendocrine system consists of the hypothalamic-pituitary-adrenal (HPA) axis and the locus caeruleus/norepinephrine-autonomic nervous system. In parallel with the evolution of the homeostasis and stress concepts from ancient Greek to modern medicine, significant advances in the field of neuroendocrinology have identified the physiologic biochemical effector molecules of the stress response. Glucocorticoids, the end-products of the HPA axis, play a fundamental role in the maintenance of both resting and stress-related homeostasis and, undoubtedly, influence the physiologic adaptive reaction of the organism against stressors. If the stress response is dysregulated in terms of magnitude and/or duration, homeostasis is turned into cacostasis with adverse effects on many vital physiologic functions, such as growth, development, metabolism, circulation, reproduction, immune response, cognition and behavior. A strong and/or long-lasting stressor may precipitate and/or cause many acute and chronic diseases. Moreover, stressors during pre-natal, post-natal or pubertal life may have a critical impact on our expressed genome. This review describes the central and peripheral components of the stress system, provides a comprehensive overview of the stress response, and discusses the role of glucocorticoids in a broad spectrum of stress-related diseases.

Introduction

All living organisms must respond to many unforeseen extrinsic or intrinsic stressful stimuli, the stressors, which constantly challenge our complex internal balance, termed homeostasis [1, 2]. The term stress is used to define a state of threatened or perceived as threatened homeostasis [3]. To respond to this threatened homeostasis, organisms have developed a highly sophisticated system,

KARGER

E-Mail karger@karger.com
www.karger.com/nim

1021–7401/14/0222–0006$39.50/0

Nicolas C. Nicolaides, MD, PhD
Division of Endocrinology and Metabolism, Clinical Research Center
Biomedical Research Foundation of the Academy of Athens
4 Soranou tou Efessiou Street, GR–11527 Athens (Greece)
E-Mail nnicolaides@bioacademy.gr

the stress system, which provides the appropriate central and peripheral neuroendocrine responses [1–3]. If these adaptive responses are inadequate, excessive or prolonged, they may have severe adverse effects on vital physiologic functions, such as growth, metabolism, circulation, reproduction and the inflammatory/immune response [3].

The stress system functions through the co-ordinated activation of the hypothalamic-pituitary-adrenal (HPA) axis and the locus caeruleus (LC)/norepinephrine (NE)-autonomic nervous system [1–3]. Glucocorticoids, the end-products of the HPA axis, are cholesterol-derived molecules that exert their pleiotropic genomic and non-genomic actions through the glucocorticoid receptor (GR), a ubiquitously expressed transcription factor, which influences the stress response substantially [4]. In this review, we describe the functional components of the stress system, provide an overview of the physical and behavioral alterations observed during the stress response, and discuss the role of glucocorticoids in the most common diseases associated with acute and chronic dysregulation of the stress system. Finally, we discuss the emerging role of the epigenetic modifications of crucial molecules involved in the adaptive response.

Historical Milestones of Stress Concepts

... he who knows things from their beginning
and origins understands them better ...
Aristotle, 4th century BC

The term stress derives from the Indo-European root 'str'. This root has been highly preserved throughout the centuries. Indeed, the ancient Greek gerund 'strangalizein', its English synonym 'to strangle' and the Latin 'strigere' have been etymologically associated with the root 'str' and have the meaning of exerted pressure [1]. Nowadays, we consider stress as a 'strangulated' balance of life.

The concepts of stress were first enunciated clearly by the ancient Greek philosophers [1, 2]. The pre-Socratic philosophers Pythagoras and Alcmaeon were the first to use the terms 'harmony' and 'isonomia', respectively, to express the dynamic balance of the cosmos or life. Pythagoras used the term 'harmony' to describe the equilibrium or balance of the universe (The harmony of the cosmos). This 'harmony' is threatened by numerous disturbing forces, while other counteracting forces tend to re-establish it. Alcmaeon of Croton termed 'isonomia' the balance of opposing forces. Empedocles of Agrigentum proposed that the four basic elements ('rhizomata' or 'racins'), earth, water, air and fire, being in dynamic opposition to one another, need to reach a balance for achieving the harmony of the cosmos (table 1) [2, 6].

Hippocrates of Cos termed health as a harmonious balance of the four humors: blood, phlegm, black and yellow bile, which correspond to the heart, the brain, the liver and the spleen, respectively. He was the first to use the term 'eucrasia' to describe the balance of the humors and subsequently proposed that their imbalance, 'dyscrasia', led to disease [2]. Hippocrates also suggested that 'eucrasia' and 'dyscrasia' have their origins in nature, and introduced the concept that 'Nature is the healer of diseases' [2]. Many years later, Epicurus spoke of 'eustatheia' or 'eustasis', which refers to the serene emotional state of a harmonious balance in a human being. The not uncommon Greek first name 'Eustathios' is a remnant of that era. Epicurus suggested that the mind could be one of these healing forces and wrote that 'ataraxia' or 'imperturbability of mind' and 'aponia' (no pain) represent desirable states in a human being [2].

During the years of Renaissance, Thomas Sydenham proposed that an individual's adaptive response to the disturbing forces that lead to systematic disharmony could result in pathologic changes. Two hundred years later, Claude Bernard suggested that the 'milieu intérieur', the internal medium that surrounds living cells, provides a steady state and 'is the pre-condition of a free and independent life' [7]. At the beginning of the 20th century, Walter Bradford Cannon coined the term 'fight or flight response', and expanded on Claude Bernard's concept of the stability of the 'milieu intérieur' to 'homeostasis' (from the Greek 'homoios', or similar, and 'stasis', or position) in order to describe the physiologic processes that maintain the steady state of the organism [2, 7]. He popularized his theories in The Wisdom of the Body, published in 1932.

Finally, Hans Hugo Bruno Selye [8], a pioneering Hungarian endocrinologist, conducted very important scientific work on the response of an organism to stressors, and described the general adaptation syndrome or stress syndrome and the diseases of adaptation. He noticed that patients with distinct disorders may present with common 'non-specific' symptoms as a common response to stressors. He borrowed the term stress from physics and defined it as 'the non-specific neuroendocrine response of the body'. Selye termed the 'General Adaptation or Stress Syndrome' as the condition occurring in severely ill patients who present with common clinical manifestations due to severe prolonged adaptation responses.

Table 1. Historical overview of stress concepts

Historical figure	Stress concept
Pythagoras (580–489 BC)	The harmony of the cosmos
Alcmaeon (c. 500 BC)	The intellect is based in the brain Health is the equipoise of opposing forces: 'Isonomia'
Empedocles (500–430 BC)	Matter consists of essential elements and qualities in opposition or alliance to one another
Hippocrates (460–375 BC)	A harmonious balance of the elements and qualities of life is health – disharmony is disease. '*Νούσων φύσεις ιητροί* = Vis medicatrix naturae'
Sceptics/Stoics Epicureans	Ataraxia (imperturbability of mind, equanimity)
Epicurus (341–270 BC)	Ataraxia (imperturbability of mind), aponia (no pain) and 'hedone' (tranquil, non-sensual pleasure) as desirable states. *'Ευστάθειος'* = good balance, Carpe diem = seize the day
Thomas Sydenham (1624–1689)	Symptoms and signs of a disease also arise from the reaction of the patients' system
Claude Bernard (1813–1878)	The 'milieu intérieur'
Walter Cannon (1871–1945)	Homeostasis/stress Bodily responses to emotions Fight or flight (and freeze) reaction
Hans Selye (1907–1982)	The general adaptation syndrome (the stress syndrome) Diseases of adaptation, distress versus eustress

Adapted from Chrousos et al. [5].

In addition to the first definition of stress, Selye coined the term 'heterostasis' (from the Greek 'heteros', or other, and 'stasis', or position) and set it to mean 'stability through change' [2, 7]. Moreover, he clarified that not all stressful conditions had adverse effects on human health; thus, 'eustress' represented those states of stress that could cause pleasant feelings and further enhance human growth and development at the emotional and intellectual level. On the other hand, he believed that 'distress' consisted of all the stressful conditions that triggered severe pathologic conditions [2]. More importantly, Selye suggested that not only the catecholamines, which are secreted by the adrenal medulla and the systemic sympathetic system, but also the adrenal cortex-derived 'corticoids' participate in the stress response [9]. He was also the first to demonstrate that glucocorticoids (which he named) exert strong anti-inflammatory effects [9]. Further to these pioneering findings, the 1950 Nobel Prize in Physiology or Medicine was jointly awarded to Edward Kendall, Philip Hench and Tadeus Reichstein for the isolation, synthesis and use of cortisone, a synthetic pre-glucocorticoid, in patients with rheumatoid arthritis.

The Stress System

The stress system has both central and peripheral components (fig. 1). The central components include: (i) the parvocellular neurons, which secrete corticotropin-releasing hormone (CRH); (ii) the neurons of the paraventricular nuclei (PVN) of the hypothalamus that secrete arginine vasopressin (AVP); (iii) the CRH neurons, which form the paragigantocellular and parabrachial nuclei of the medulla and the LC, and (iv) other neural groups in the medulla and pons (LC/NE system) mostly secreting NE. The peripheral components include: (i) the neuroendocrine HPA axis; (ii) the efferent systemic sympathetic-adrenomedullary systems, and (iii) components functioning under the control of the parasympathetic system [10].

The central and peripheral components of the stress system have many sites of interaction with other systems at multiple levels [1, 2, 10, 11] (fig. 2). Indeed, activation of CRH neurons activates the LC/NE system and vice versa. In addition to interactions between the two central components of the stress system themselves, the stress system activates the mesocortical and the mesolimbic dopaminergic reward system, while it receives inhibitory input from the

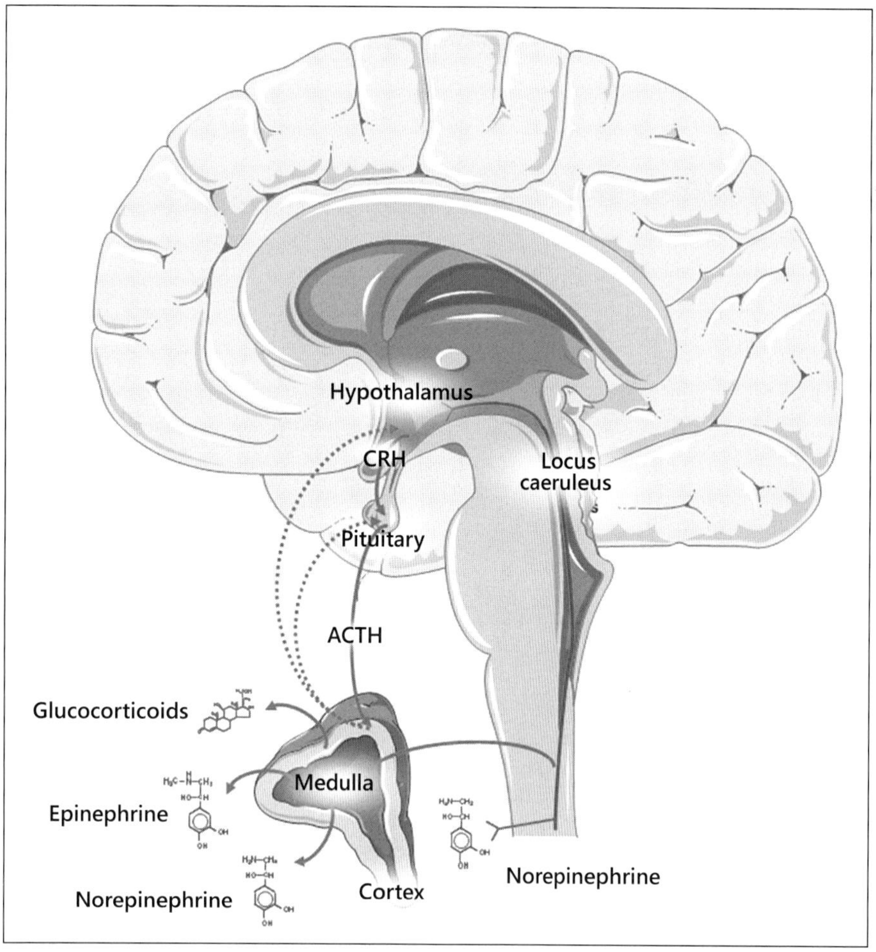

Color version available online

Fig. 1. The stress system. Modified from Chrousos [12].

latter systems [2, 10, 11]. The stress system also activates the central nucleus of the amygdala, which participates in the generation of fear and/or anger; upon activation, the central nucleus of the amygdala stimulates the stress system, forming a positive regulatory feedback loop with it [2, 10, 11]. The PVN of hypothalamus communicates with the arcuate nucleus through CRH neurons that induce the release of α-melanocyte-stimulating hormone and β-endorphin from the pro-opiomelanocortin-containing neurons in the arcuate nucleus. These two molecules both inhibit the activity of the CRH and LC/NE systems. Moreover, the two components of the stress system appear to respond to many neurochemical modulators, such as serotonin and acetylcholine, which are acutely stimulatory, and γ-aminobutyric acid and benzodiazepines, which are inhibitory to CRH neurons and the LC/NE system [2, 10, 11]. Finally, the neuropeptide Y, leptin and substance P have been recently shown to play an important role in the regulation of stress system activity [11].

Significant progress in the evolving field of neuroendocrinology uncovered the key molecules involved in the complex molecular pathways of the above central and peripheral anatomical loci responsible for the generation and regulation of the stress response. CRH, AVP and NE play the role of bona fide neurotransmitters primarily – but not exclusively – in the CNS, whereas NE, epinephrine and the glucocorticoids, which will be discussed in a separate section of this review article, are considered to be the final effector molecules of the peripheral stress system.

The HPA Axis

The HPA axis consists of stimulatory signals and negative feedback loops that regulate its activity. This neuroendocrine axis is composed of three distinct anatomical loci: the PVN of the hypothalamus, the pituitary gland and the adrenal cortices (fig. 1). A broad spectrum of

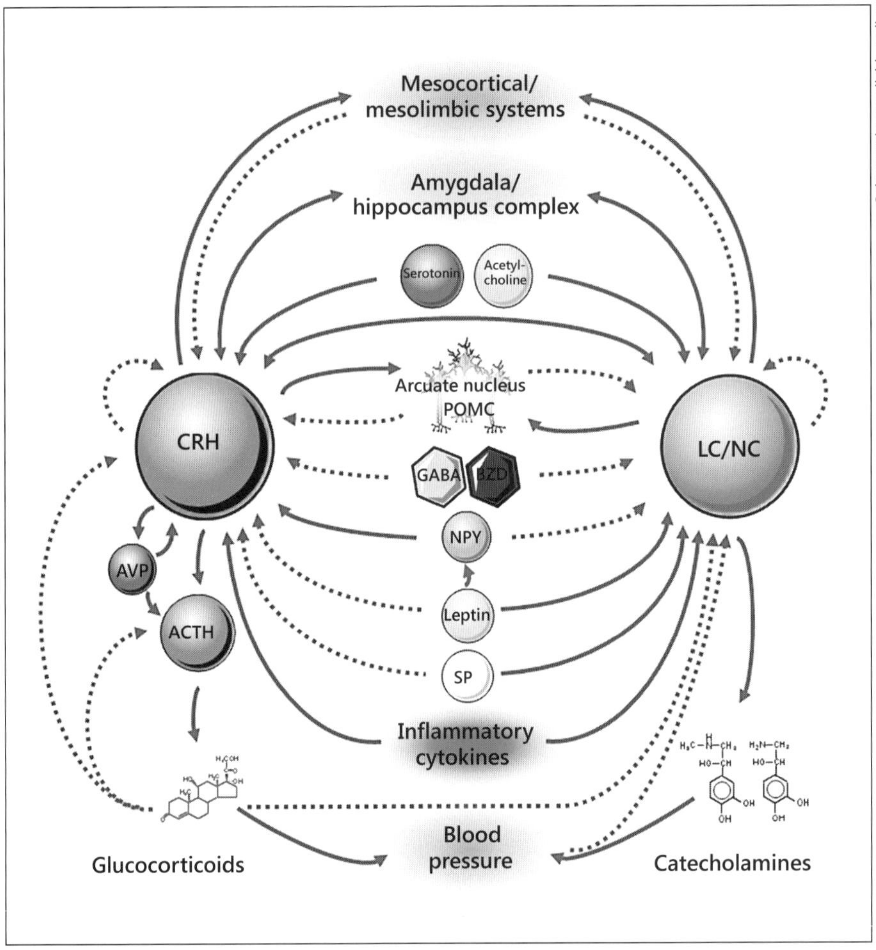

Fig. 2. Schematic representation of the central and peripheral components of the stress system, their functional interrelations and their interactions with other homeostatic systems and molecules involved in the stress response. Activation is represented by solid lines and inhibition by dashed lines. POMC = Pro-opiomelanocortin; GABA = γ-aminobutyric acid; BZD = benzodiazepine; NPY = neuropeptide Y; SP = substance P. Modified from Chrousos and Gold [2].

stressors trigger the synthesis and secretion of CRH and AVP by a group of neurons located in the PVN of the hypothalamus [12, 13]. CRH, through the hypophysial portal system, reaches the anterior lobe of the pituitary gland and binds to its cognate G-protein-coupled receptor leading to the production and release of adrenocorticotropic hormone (ACTH) into the systemic circulation [14, 15]. Upon binding to its transmembrane G-protein-coupled receptor of the adrenocortical cells of the *zona fasciculata*, ACTH induces the activity of proteins and the expression of genes implicated in the biosynthetic pathway of glucocorticoids (cortisol in humans, corticosterone in rodents) [16]. Moreover, ACTH regulates adrenal androgen secretion by the *zona reticularis*, and participates in the control of aldosterone secretion by the *zona glomerulosa*.

Glucocorticoids, the end-products of the HPA axis, are steroid hormones with pleiotropic effects in almost all tissues and organs. These molecules regulate the basal activity of the HPA axis and terminate the stress response by acting mainly at the hypothalamus and the pituitary gland, thereby forming negative feedback loops on the secretion of CRH and ACTH, respectively. These negative feedback mechanisms, especially in the case of ACTH, appear to also be mediated by non-genomic rapid glucocorticoid actions [17].

Genomic and Non-Genomic Glucocorticoid Actions

Glucocorticoids are cholesterol-derived hormones, which play a fundamental role in the maintenance of resting and stress-related homeostasis. These molecules are involved in the maintenance of proper cardiovascular tone, regulate the intermediary metabolism primarily through catabolic actions in the liver, muscle and adipose tissue, and influence substantially the quantity and quality of the inflammatory and immune response. Furthermore, vital functions, such as reproduction, growth, be-

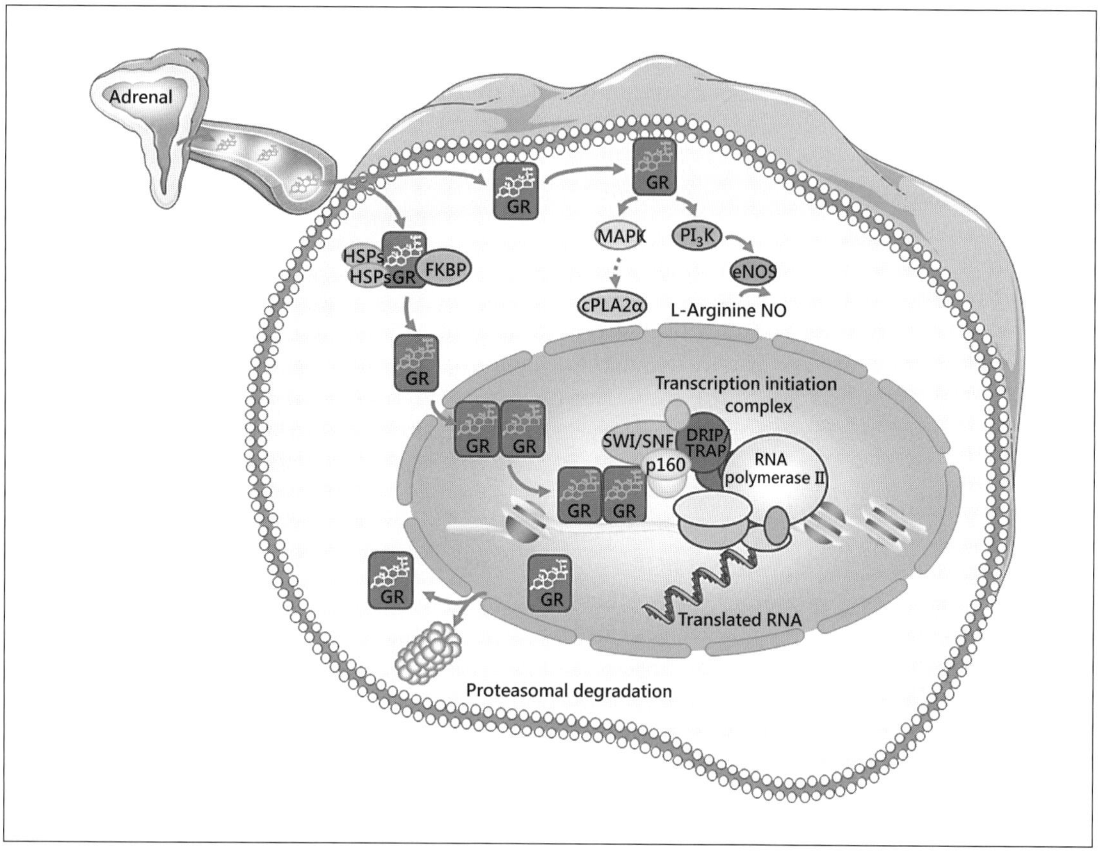

Color version available online

Fig. 3. Molecular pathways of genomic and non-genomic glucocorticoid actions. HSP = Heat shock proteins; FKBP = immunophilins; p160 = nuclear receptor co-activators p160; SWI/SNF = switching/sucrose non-fermenting complex; DRIP/TRAP = vitamin D receptor-interacting protein/thyroid hormone receptor-associated protein complex; MAPK = mitogen-activated protein kinases; cPLA2α = cytosolic phospholipase A2 alpha; PI_3K = phosphatidylinositol 3-kinase; eNOS = endothelial nitric oxide synthetase; NO = nitric oxide.

havior, cognition, cell proliferation and survival are under the control of genomic and non-genomic glucocorticoid actions [3, 4, 18]. Glucocorticoids also contribute to water and electrolyte homeostasis. All these are essential life functions of glucocorticoids and are mediated by an intracellular, ubiquitously expressed protein, the human GR (hGR), which belongs to the steroid receptor family of the nuclear receptor superfamily of transcription factors [19].

In humans, the *hGR* gene is located on the short arm of chromosome 5 and consists of 10 exons [19]. Exon 1 forms the 5′-untranslated region, whereas the rest of the exons encode the protein. The alternative use of two distinct exons, 9α and 9β, gives rise to two main protein isoforms, the hGRα and the hGRβ [18, 19]. Lu and Cidlowski [20] showed that the translation of hGRα mRNA could start from eight alternative sites through ribosomal leaky scanning or ribosomal shunting producing eight functionally distinct hGRα protein isoforms. Since hGRβ mRNA translation is initiated by the same 5′ termini, it is possible that the same translation mechanisms could also generate eight different hGRβ proteins [18]. The total of sixteen hGRα and hGRβ isoforms may potentially form 256 homo- or hetero-dimers to transduce the glucocorticoid signal within the target cells, turning the simplified glucocorticoid signaling pathway into a highly stochastic system.

Within the target cell, the unliganded hGRα is primarily localized in the cytoplasm of cells forming a large multi-protein complex with the chaperon heat shock proteins 90 and 70, as well as other proteins, such as the immunophilins (fig. 3). Upon ligand-binding, hGRα dissociates from the multi-protein complex, translocates into the nucleus and interacts, as a homo- or hetero-dimer, with specific DNA sequences, the glucocorticoid response elements (GREs) in the promoter regions of target genes, influencing their transcription rate in a positive or negative way. Following binding to GREs, the receptor undergoes further conformational changes that lead to serial and co-ordinated recruitment of nuclear receptor co-activators [p160, p300/CREB-binding protein (CBP) and p300/CBP-associated factor] and chromatin-remodeling complexes (switching/sucrose non-fermenting complex and vitamin D receptor-interacting protein/thyroid hormone receptor-associated protein complex). This molecular complex influences the activity of the RNA polymerase II and its ancillary factors, thereby facilitating initiation of the transcriptional process of numerous glucocorticoid-responsive genes [19] (fig. 3).

Alternatively, gene expression can be modulated by the ligand-activated hGRα in a GRE-independent fashion. Several studies have shown that hGRα physically interacted, possibly as a monomer, with other core transcription factors, such as the NF-κB, activator protein-1 (c-Fos/c-Jun, AP-1), p53 and signal transducers and activators of transcription (STATs), thus increasing or inhibiting their transcriptional activity [18, 19]. Importantly, the major anti-inflammatory and immunosuppressive effects of glucocorticoids appear to be mediated mostly by the interaction of the activated hGRα with the pro-inflammatory transcription factors NF-κB and AP-1.

Interestingly, it was recently shown that the transcription factor 'circadian locomotor output cycle kaput' (CLOCK), which forms a heterodimer with its partner brain-muscle Arnt-like protein 1 (BMAL1), is a novel partner of GR and catalyzes the acetylation of lysine residues within the hinge region of the receptor, thus leading to decreased sensitivity to glucocorticoids. These in vitro studies have also demonstrated that the heterodimer CLOCK/BMAL1 behaves as a negative regulator of hGRα in peripheral target tissues, and antagonizes the physiologic actions of fluctuating cortisol [21–24]. Further in vivo and ex vivo studies demonstrated that CLOCK-mediated acetylation of hGRα was higher in the morning (when circulating cortisol concentrations are elevated), leading to decreased tissue sensitivity to glucocorticoids. In contrast, hGRα was less acetylated by CLOCK at night (when cortisol concentrations reach their nadir), which resulted in increased sensitivity of tissues to glucocorticoids [25]. The CLOCK system and the HPA axis communicate with one another at multiple signaling levels; therefore, any conditions that disrupt their molecular communication may lead to the development of the metabolic syndrome [22–24]. Indeed, night-shift workers and people frequently exposed to jet lag are at an increased risk for developing symptoms and signs of chronic hypercortisolemia, such as central obesity, insulin resistance, dyslipidemia and hypertension, which represent the cardinal clinical manifestations of metabolic syndrome [22–24].

In addition to the above-described genomic actions, accumulating evidence suggests that glucocorticoids can induce some of their pleiotropic actions within seconds or minutes. Apart from their short time frame, these glucocorticoid actions do not require hGRα-mediated transcription/translation, and thus are referred to as 'non-genomic', and can occur in various systems, including the neuroendocrine, cardiovascular and immune systems [26–29]. Representative examples of non-genomic glucocorticoid actions are: (i) the immediate suppression of ACTH secretion from the anterior pituitary by glucocorticoids [30]; (ii) the glucocorticoid-induced rapid increase in the frequency of excitatory post-synaptic potentials in the hippocampus [31]; (iii) the rapid and transient decrease in blood pressure associated with a concomitant increase in coronary and cerebral blood flow in patients with myocardial infarction or stroke [32], and (iv) the rapid inhibition of T cell receptor signaling through disruption of the T cell receptor complex [33]. These actions are thought to be mediated by membrane-localized GRs, which, upon ligand binding, trigger the activation of kinase signaling cascades, such as the mitogen-activated protein kinase or the phosphatidylinositol 3-kinase pathways [26–29]. Although the downstream events of non-genomic glucocorticoid signal transduction have been partially elucidated, the origin and membrane localization mechanism(s) of the membrane GR still remain an enigma.

The LC/NE, Systemic Sympathetic, Adrenomedullary and Parasympathetic Nervous Systems

The sympathetic and parasympathetic systems represent the two functional components of the autonomic nervous system and influence the activity of many vital physiologic systems, such as respiratory, cardiovascular, renal, gastrointestinal, neuroendocrine and others. The sympathetic system plays an important role through the adrenal medulla in the 'fight or flight reaction' by secreting all circulating epinephrine and some of the NE [11]. On the other hand, the parasympathetic system antagonizes or assists sympathetic functions by increasing or withdrawing its activity, respectively [10, 11].

To transmit the neural signal, the sympathetic and parasympathetic systems employ the well-known neurotransmitters acetylcholine and NE, numerous neuropeptides, as well as lipid mediators of inflammation, adenosine triphosphate or nitric oxide [11].

The Adaptive Response to Stress

When homeostasis is threatened or perceived as threatened by a stressor, the stress system is activated through two waves of serial hormonal secretion providing the adaptive response. The first wave begins within seconds and involves: (i) increased release of epinephrine and NE from the sympathetic nervous system; (ii) secretion of hypothalamic CRH into the hypophysial portal system and subsequent enhanced release of ACTH; (iii) decreased release of hypothalamic gonadotropin-releasing hormone (GnRH) followed by decreased secretion of follicle-stimulating hormone (FSH) and luteinizing hormone (LH) from the anterior pituitary, and (iv) enhanced secretion of pituitary-derived prolactin and growth hormone (GH), and increased release of glycogen from the pancreas [34].

A second wave of hormonal secretion occurs more slowly and involves the glucocorticoids. All these stress-mediated hormonal changes during both waves are translated in cellular end-effects. The hormones involved in the first wave signal through GPCRs and rapid second messenger pathways. By contrast, glucocorticoids activate the GR, a transcription factor that needs more time from at least 20 min to hours and even days to complete the appropriate molecular scenario.

However, mounting evidence suggests that many of the non-genomic glucocorticoid actions are undoubtedly involved in the acute phase of the stress response [35, 36]. Not only do glucocorticoids bind to membrane GRs, but they also trigger the mineralocorticoid receptor (MR), another member of the steroid hormone receptor family of transcription factors, which is evolutionarily related to the GR. It seems that glucocorticoids, even at lower concentrations than those activating the GR, bind to membrane or cytoplasmic MRs and increase the activity of multiple kinases involved in distinct signal transduction cascades. Both the GR and MR play important roles in glutamatergic neurotransmission (fig. 4).

During stress, increased concentrations of glucocorticoids activate post-synaptic membrane-localized GRs, which, through the c-AMP-protein kinase A (PKA) pathway, induce the production and release of the retrograde molecules anandamide and 2-arachidonoylglycerol. The latter activate the cannabinoid receptors type 1, located at the membrane of pre-synaptic neurons, which finally inhibit the secretion of glutamate-containing vesicles [35–37]. On the other hand, pre- and post-synaptic membrane MRs appear to facilitate glutamatergic transmission. Presynaptically, glucocorticoids bind to membrane MRs, which, in turn, induce the activation of the extracellular signal-regulated kinase cascade, leading to glutamate release in the synaptic space. Simultaneously, the post-synaptic activation of membrane MRs by glucocorticoids results in the inhibition of potassium I_A-currents, and facilitates the membrane diffusion of AMPA receptors [35, 36]. The above-discussed examples show convincingly that glucocorticoids, acting through the classic transcription factor GR, also participate in even the early non-genomic molecular events underlying the adaptive response.

Activation of the stress system through the above neuroendocrine mechanisms leads to a series of behavioral and physical adaptation changes that increase acutely the chances for survival [1–4, 10, 11]. Therefore, organisms may present with alertness, increased arousal, vigilance, improved cognition, focused attention, as well as euphoria, enhanced analgesia, suppression of feeding and inhibition of reproductive function. In addition to behavioral alterations, physical adaptation changes occur under stressful conditions. Thus, oxygen and nutrients are redirected to the CNS and the stressed body site(s) through a high respiratory rate, increased cardiovascular tone and a shift of intermediary metabolism towards catabolism. Moreover, organisms activate detoxification processes for any unnecessary metabolic products from the stress-related reactions [10]. Concurrently, organisms 'switch on' restraining mechanisms during stress, which prevent an over-response from the stress system. If they fail to control stress-related adaptive changes, the stress response may become excessive, prolonged and maladaptive and may, thus, contribute to the development of acute or chronic pathologic conditions.

Stress System Disorders

Everything in moderation
Inscription at the Oracle of Delphi

Homeostasis is effectively achieved through normal basal activity of the stress system and the appropriate quantity and quality of the stress response to stressors [1, 2]. These parameters are *sine qua non* for human health.

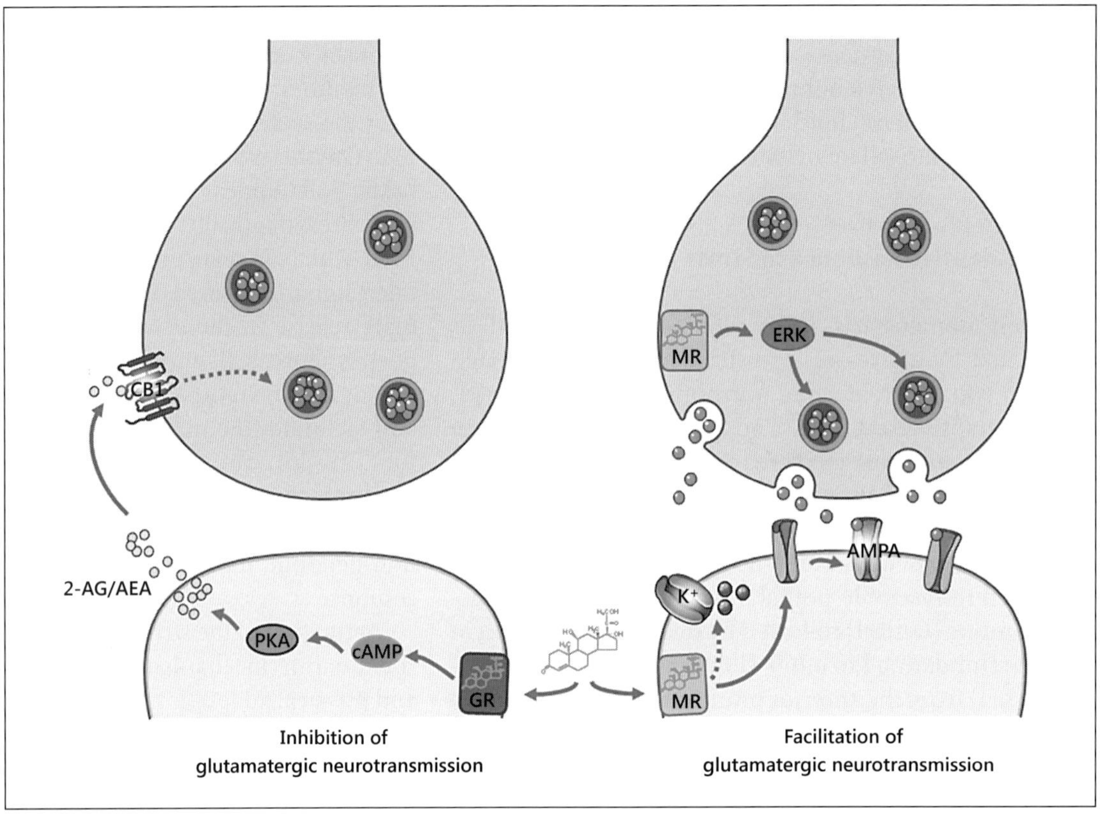

Color version available online

Fig. 4. Inhibition and facilitation of glutamatergic neurotransmission through membrane GRs and MRs, respectively. cAMP = Cyclic-AMP; 2-AG = 2-arachidonoylglycerol; AEA = anandamide; CB1 = cannabinoid receptor type 1; K^+ = potassium; AMPA = α-amino-3-hydroxy-5-methyl-4-isoxazolepropionic acid receptor; ERK = extracellular signal-regulated kinase. Modified from Groeneweg et al. [35].

By contrast, if the stress system has low or high basal activity and/or excessive or prolonged responsiveness to stressful stimuli, homeostasis is turned into cacostasis with many adverse consequences on physiologic biologic functions, leading to the development of acute or chronic pathologic conditions.

Acute and Chronic Stress System Disorders

Stress may precipitate acute or chronic disorders in humans with susceptible genetic loci and/or epigenetic modifications in several genes [1–4, 10–12, 38]. Under acute stress, individuals may present with allergic conditions (asthma, eczema or urticaria), or complaint for migraines and/or gastrointestinal symptoms, such as abdominal pain, indigestion, diarrhea and constipation. Of note, the frequency of panic attacks and psychotic episodes is higher during acute stress. The molecular basis of these stress-mediated conditions can be attributed to acutely increased secretion of CRH, which exerts its effects through signaling in vulnerable end organs [39–43]. On the other hand, a long-lasting stress response may cause excessive release and prolonged effects of the major effector molecules of the stress system, including CRH, cortisol and NE, on vital neuroendocrine and metabolic axes leading to the development of a broad spectrum of metabolic and/or neuropsychiatric disorders [1, 4, 18, 39–43].

Chronic stress exerts inhibitory effects on the growth axis. Chronically increased circulating glucocorticoids suppress the secretion of GH from the pituitary and inhibit insulin-like growth factor I actions at its target tissues, possibly through interaction of the c-jun/c-fos heterodimer with the ligand-activated hGR [44–46]. Furthermore, CRH increases the levels of hypothalamic somatostatin, a known inhibitor of GH secretion. These mechanisms may explain the delayed or arrested growth in children with Cushing syndrome [45, 47]. Another example of stress-mediated inhibition of growth is the 'psychosocial short stature' in children or adolescents who experienced physical or psychological maltreatment. These children have typically decreased levels of GH, which return to within a normal range a few days after they are separated from the stressful environment [48, 49].

Prolonged activation of the stress system leads to decreased synthesis of thyroid-stimulating hormone due to increased concentrations of CRH-induced somatostatin, which in turn suppresses both thyroid-releasing hormone (TRH) and thyroid-stimulating hormone (TSH). Furthermore, elevated circulating concentrations of glucocorticoids inhibit the activity of the enzyme 5-deiodinase that converts inactive thyroxine to the biologically active triiodothyronine in peripheral target tissues (the 'euthyroid sick' syndrome) [50].

The hypothalamic-pituitary-gonadal axis is strongly influenced at multiple levels by both CRH and glucocorticoids [51]. CRH inhibits the secretion of GnRH from the hypothalamus [52, 53], while glucocorticoids suppress the activity of the reproductive axis by decreasing secretion of GnRH, follicle-stimulating hormone/luteinizing hormone and gonadal steroids [52–55]. Representative examples of stress-mediated suppression of the gonadal axis are highly trained runners and ballet dancers, who may present with suppression of gonadal function due to chronic activation of the HPA axis [56, 57].

Individuals under chronic stress are more susceptible to specific infections and autoimmune disorders caused by the glucocorticoid- and catecholamine-induced switch from Th1 to Th2 [11, 12, 38, 40, 41]. Indeed, chronically stressed individuals may have persistent infections with *Helicobacter pylori*, *Mycobacterium tuberculosis* and the common cold viruses. Moreover, the stress-induced Th1 to Th2 switch increases the risk for certain autoimmune disorders, such as systemic lupus erythematosus, Graves disease, and some allergic conditions [1].

Stress System and Non-Communicable Diseases

At present, our society is plagued by complex multifactorial non-communicable diseases, including obesity/metabolic syndrome and its detrimental cardiovascular complications, as well as depression, anxiety and insomnia. All these pathologic conditions are associated with an excessive or long-lasting stress response to a variety of external or internal stressors.

The pathogenesis of metabolic syndrome is closely associated with chronic hypersecretion of stress system mediators, such as cortisol, NE, epinephrine, immune CRH and IL-6, which increase the secretion of insulin and decrease the release of GH and sex steroids, ultimately leading to visceral fat accumulation, and loss of muscle mass (sarcopenia) and bone mass (osteoporosis) [58, 59]. The resultant visceral obesity and sarcopenia are closely associated with other cardinal clinical manifestations of the metabolic syndrome, such as dyslipidemia, hypertension and type 2 diabetes mellitus. Moreover, elevated concentrations of IL-6, among other cytokines secreted by inflamed adipose tissue, and chronic hypercortisolism contribute to stimulation of acute-phase reaction and blood hypercoagulation. All these adverse factors may lead to endothelial dysfunction and atherosclerotic cardiovascular disease [1, 58, 59].

In addition to the metabolic syndrome, stress participates in the pathogenesis of major depression [60–62]. Major depression is a heterogeneous disorder with two main subtypes: melancholic and atypical depression. Patients with melancholic depression have a hyperactive stress system and may present with anxiety, guilt, fear, low self-esteem, insomnia and loss of appetite. They also have hypersecretion of hypothalamic CRH, as evidenced by elevated 24-hour urinary cortisol excretion, decreased ACTH responses to exogenous CRH administration, and elevated concentrations of CRH in their cerebrospinal fluid throughout the 24-hour period. Furthermore, the concentrations of NE in cerebrospinal fluid are continuously elevated, even during sleep. In contradistinction to melancholic depression, atypical depression is characterized by lethargy, fatigue, hypersomnia and hyperphagia, which are associated with downregulation of the HPA axis of central origin.

All the above-discussed chronic non-communicable disorders of modern societies are associated with maladaptive stress responses and their origins lie deep in the evolutionary process of human beings [1, 4, 63]. Indeed, our ancestors faced numerous environmental stressors, including starvation, dehydration, infectious diseases, threatening adversaries, dangers and injuries, which applied selective pressures upon genes implicated in the adaptive stress response. This genomic selection obviously favored those individuals who were efficient in coping with the above stressful stimuli.

Today, the same selected gene networks, subserving functions important for human survival and species preservation, must encode effector molecules involved in the 'contemporary' adaptive stress response to address the same types of stressors, but in different quantities and

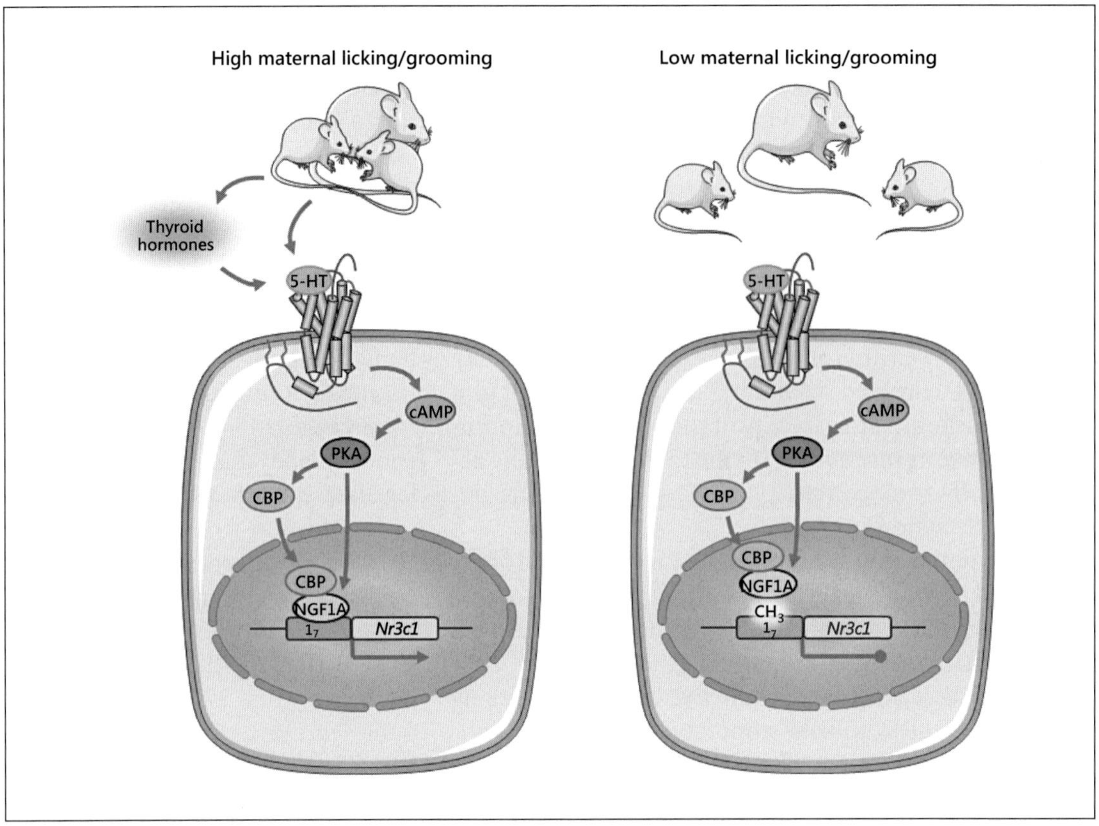

Fig. 5. Molecular mechanisms linking maternal licking/grooming with hippocampal GR expression. cAMP = Cyclic-AMP; NGFIA = nerve growth factor-inducible A; *Nr3c1* = nuclear receptor subfamily 3, group C, member 1 (GR) gene. Modified from Champagne [68].

Table 2. Gene networks subserving functions important for human survival and species preservation, which may produce pathology in contemporary Western societies

Response to survival threat	Selective advantage	Contemporary diseases
Combat starvation	Energy conservation	Obesity
Combat dehydration	Fluid and electrolyte conservation	Hypertension
Combat infectious diseases	Potent immune reaction	Autoimmunity/allergy
Anticipate adversaries	Arousal/fear	Anxiety/insomnia
Minimize exposure to danger	Withdrawal from danger	Depression
Prevent tissue strain and injury	Retain tissue integrity and reserve	Pain and fatigue syndromes

Adapted from Chrousos and Kino [4].

contexts. For example, an excess of calories leads to obesity, since the adaptive stress response has been programmed to cope with food deficiency, not excess. Thus, the gene networks presented in table 2 are now accepted to be responsible for most of the contemporary diseases of Western societies.

The Stress System in the Epigenetic Era

Interactions between genetic and environmental factors have been confirmed by many epidemiological studies [64]. However, the molecular mechanisms through which the environment acts to switch genes 'on' and 'off' remain incompletely elucidated and are currently under intense investigation.

Almost 30 years ago, a brief report published by Meaney et al. [65] provided the first evidence of an association between post-natal pup handling and GR levels within the hippocampus. In their pioneering work, they compared rats exposed to maternal handling with non-handled ones. They demonstrated that handled rats had significantly increased protein levels of GR expressed in the hippocampus compared with the non-handled rats [65]. At that time, two possible mechanisms were proposed to explain these effects: (i) elevated protein levels of GR per cell, and (ii) increased post-natal neurogenesis in the hippocampus in the handled rats. These results set the stage for further molecular and cellular studies. Thus, it was later shown that handling could increase the concentrations of plasma thyroid hormones (thyroxine and triiodothyronine) [66], and that both handling and thyroid hormones might boost serotonin (5-HT) turnover in hippocampal neurons [67].

Further studies determined the molecules involved in the serotonin-mediated GR expression [68] (fig. 5). Upon binding to the 5-HT receptor, handling-induced serotonin molecules trigger the production of c-AMP and the subsequent activation of PKA. The latter facilitates – directly or indirectly through CBP – the binding of the transcription factor nerve growth factor-inducible factor A (NGFI-A) to a specific region of exon 1_7 of the *Nr3c1* gene inducing the expression of GR within the hippocampus. The procedure of handling has been shown to correspond to increased maternal licking/grooming [69].

Subsequent studies demonstrated that high maternal licking/grooming resulted in elevated thyroid hormone levels, enhanced serotonin signaling and increased binding of NGFI-A to the *Nr3c1* 1_7 promoter [70]. By contrast, low maternal licking/grooming led to low GR expression that was attributed to increased hippocampal cytosine methylation of the *Nr3c1* 1_7 promoter, an epigenetic modification that obviously altered gene expression without any changes in the underlying DNA sequence [71]. The application of epigenetics research in humans showed a clear association of childhood abuse with increased *Nr3c1* 1_7 methylation at the NGFI-A binding sites [72].

In addition to GR, other studies have investigated stress-induced epigenetic modifications of genes involved in the stress response. Among them, the *Crh*, glial-derived neurotrophic factor *(Gdnf)*, brain-derived neurotrophic factor *(Bdnf)* and AVP *(Avp)* genes were studied exclusively in animal models [73]. Although all these epigenetic modifications are persistent and can be present in the next generation, recent evidence suggests that drugs altering DNA methylation/histone modifications can reverse the effects of early life experience in adulthood [74]. Thus, the emerging field of behavioral epigenetics will be at the epicenter of stress research and will undoubtedly provide a significant contribution to our conceptualization of the impact of early-life events on the quality of adult life [75].

Conclusions

We now know the central and peripheral components of the stress system, the physiologic biochemical effectors that mediate the behavioral and physical changes during the stress response, and the molecular mechanisms through which stress-induced neuroendocrine changes are translated to target tissue effects. Distress is a major factor in the pathogenetic mechanisms of almost all disorders. Moreover, our lifestyles and environment in modern societies seem to be particularly permissive for allostasis. The picture became more complicated when we realized that early stressful life experiences leave deep traces in our expressed genome. It is imperative to develop effective strategies of stress management to decrease the incidence and alleviate the symptoms and consequences of stress system disorders. Although there remains much to learn about stress-mediated pathogenetic mechanisms, it is certain that less distress improves the quality and increases the length of our lives.

Acknowledgments

This work was supported by: (i) the European Union (European Social Fund – ESF) and Greek national funds through the Operational Program 'Education and Lifelong Learning' of the National Strategic Reference Framework (NSRF) – Research Funding Program: THALIS – University of Athens, Athens, Greece; and (ii) the intramural program of the *Eunice Kennedy Shriver* National Institute of Child Health and Human Development, National Institutes of Health, Bethesda, Md., USA.

All figures were prepared using image vectors from Servier Medical Art (www.servier.com), licensed under the Creative Commons Attribution 3.0 Unported License (http://creativecommons.org/license/by/3.0/).

References

1 Chrousos GP: Stress and disorders of the stress system. Nat Rev Endocrinol 2009;5: 374–381.
2 Chrousos GP, Gold PW: The concepts of stress and stress system disorders: overview of physical and behavioral homeostasis. JAMA 1992;267:1244–1252.
3 Charmandari E, Tsigos C, Chrousos GP: Endocrinology of the stress response. Annu Rev Physiol 2005;67:259–284.
4 Chrousos GP, Kino T: Glucocorticoid action networks and complex psychiatric and/or somatic disorders. Stress 2007;10:213–219.
5 Chrousos GP, Loriaux DL, Gold PW (eds): Mechanisms of Physical and Emotional Stress: Advances in Experimental Medicine and Biology. New York, Plenum Press, 1988, vol 245.
6 Kontopoulou TD, Marketos SG: Homeostasis: the ancient Greek origin of a modern scientific principle. Hormones 2002;1:124–125.
7 Fink G: Stress: definition and history; in Squire LR (ed): Encyclopedia of Neuroscience. Oxford, Academic Press, 2009, pp 549–555, vol 9.
8 Selye H: A syndrome produced by diverse nocuous agents. Nature 1936;138:32.
9 Szabo S, Tache Y, Somogyi A: The legacy of Hans Selye and the origins of stress research: a retrospective 75 years after his landmark brief 'letter' to the editor of *Nature*. Stress 2012;15:472–478.
10 Charmandari E, Kino T, Souvatzoglou E, Chrousos GP: Pediatric stress: hormonal mediators and human development. Horm Res 2003;59:161–179.
11 Chrousos GP: Stressors, stress, and neuroendocrine integration of the adaptive response: the 1997 Hans Selye Memorial Lecture. Ann NY Acad Sci 1998;851:311–335.
12 Chrousos GP: The hypothalamic-pituitary-adrenal axis and immune-mediated inflammation. N Engl J Med 1995;332:1351–1362.
13 Chrousos GP, Calabrese JR, Avgerinos P, Kling MA, Rubinow D, Oldfield EH, et al: Corticotropin releasing factor: basic studies and clinical applications. Prog Neuropsychopharmacol Biol Psychiatry 1985;9:349–359.
14 Calogero AE, Bernardini R, Gold PW, Chrousos GP: Regulation of rat hypothalamic corticotropin-releasing hormone secretion in vitro: potential clinical implications. Adv Exp Med Biol 1988;245:167–181.
15 Smith MA, Kling MA, Whitfield HJ, Brandt HA, Demitrack MA, Geracioti TD, Chrousos GP, Gold PW: Corticotropin-releasing hormone: from endocrinology to psychobiology. Horm Res 1989;31:66–71.
16 Bornstein SR, Chrousos GP: Clinical review 104: Adrenocorticotropin (ACTH)- and non-ACTH-mediated regulation of the adrenal cortex: neural and immune inputs. J Clin Endocrinol Metab 1999;84:1729–1736.
17 Hammes SR, Levin ER: Extranuclear steroid receptors: nature and actions. Endocr Rev 2007;28:726–741.
18 Chrousos GP, Kino T: Intracellular glucocorticoid signaling: a formerly simple system turns stochastic. Sci STKE 2005;2005:pe48.
19 Nicolaides NC, Galata Z, Kino T, Chrousos GP, Charmandari E: The human glucocorticoid receptor: molecular basis of biologic function. Steroids 2010;75:1–12.
20 Lu NZ, Cidlowski JA: Translational regulatory mechanisms generate N-terminal glucocorticoid receptor isoforms with unique transcriptional target genes. Mol Cell 2005;18: 331–342.
21 Nader N, Chrousos GP, Kino T: Circadian rhythm transcription factor CLOCK regulates the transcriptional activity of the glucocorticoid receptor by acetylating its hinge region lysine cluster: potential physiological implications. FASEB J 2009;23:1572–1583.
22 Nader N, Chrousos GP, Kino T: Interactions of the circadian CLOCK system and the HPA axis. Trends Endocrinol Metab 2010;21:277–286.
23 Kino T, Chrousos GP: Acetylation-mediated epigenetic regulation of glucocorticoid receptor activity: circadian rhythm-associated alterations of glucocorticoid actions in target tissues. Mol Cell Endocrinol 2011;336:23–30.
24 Kino T, Chrousos GP: Circadian CLOCK-mediated regulation of target-tissue sensitivity to glucocorticoids: implications for cardiometabolic diseases. Endocr Dev 2011;20:116–126.
25 Charmandari E, Chrousos GP, Lambrou GI, Pavlaki A, Koide H, Ng SSM, Kino T: Peripheral CLOCK regulates target-tissue glucocorticoid receptor transcriptional activity in a circadian fashion in man. PLoS ONE 2011; 6:e25612.
26 Ayroldi E, Cannarile L, Migliorati G, Nocentini G, Delfino DV, Riccardi C: Mechanisms of the anti-inflammatory effects of glucocorticoids: genomic and nongenomic interference with MAPK signaling pathways. FASEB J 2012;26:4805–4820.
27 Song IH, Buttgereit F: Non-genomic glucocorticoid effects to provide the basis for new drug developments. Mol Cell Endocrinol 2006;246:142–146.
28 Lee SR, Kim HK, Youm JB, Dizon LA, Song IS, Jeong SH, Seo DY, Ko KS, Rhee BD, Kim N, Han J: Non-genomic effect of glucocorticoids on cardiovascular system. Pflügers Arch 2012;464:549–559.
29 Bellavance MA, Rivest S: The neuroendocrine control of the innate immune system in health and brain diseases. Immunol Rev 2012;248: 36–55.
30 Hinz B, Hirschelmann R: Rapid non-genomic feedback effects of glucocorticoids on CRF-induced ACTH secretion in rats. Pharm Res 2000;17:1273–1277.
31 Karst H, Berger S, Turiault M, Tronche F, Schütz G, Joëls M: Mineralocorticoid receptors are indispensable for nongenomic modulation of hippocampal glutamate transmission by corticosterone. Proc Natl Acad Sci USA 2005;102:19204–19207.
32 Hafezi-Moghadam A, Simoncini T, Yang Z, Limbourg FP, Plumier JC, Rebsamen MC, Hsieh CM, Chui DS, Thomas KL, Prorock AJ, Laubach VE, Moskowitz MA, French BA, Ley K, Liao JK: Acute cardiovascular protective effects of corticosteroids are mediated by non-transcriptional activation of endothelial nitric oxide synthase. Nat Med 2002;8:473–479.
33 Löwenberg M, Verhaar AP, Bilderbeek J, Marle J, Buttgereit F, Peppelenbosch MP, van Deventer SJ, Hommes DW: Glucocorticoids cause rapid dissociation of a T-cell-receptor-associated protein complex containing LCK and FYN. EMBO Rep 2006;7:1023–1029.
34 Sapolsky RM, Romero LM, Munck AU: How do glucocorticoids influence stress responses? Integrating permissive, suppressive, stimulatory, and preparative actions. Endocr Rev 2000;21:55–89.
35 Groeneweg FL, Karst H, de Kloet ER, Joëls M: Rapid non-genomic effects of corticosteroids and their role in the central stress response. J Endocrinol 2011;209:153–167.
36 Prager EM, Johnson LR: Stress at the synapse: signal transduction mechanisms of adrenal steroids at neuronal membranes. Sci Signal 2009;2:re5.
37 Tasker JG, Di S, Malcher-Lopes R: Minireview: rapid glucocorticoid signaling via membrane-associated receptors. Endocrinology 2006;147:5549–5556.
38 Chrousos GP: The stress response and immune function: clinical implications – the 1999 Novera H. Spector lecture. Ann NY Acad Sci 2000;917:38–67.
39 Karalis K, Sano H, Redwine J, Listwak S, Wilder RL, Chrousos GP: Autocrine or paracrine inflammatory actions of corticotropin-releasing hormone in vivo. Science 1991;254: 421–423.
40 Elenkov IJ, Chrousos GP: Stress hormones, Th1/Th2-patterns, pro/anti- inflammatory cytokines and susceptibility to disease. Trends Endocrinol Metab 1999;10:359–368.
41 Elenkov IJ, Kvetnansky R, Hashiramoto A, Bakalov VK, Link AA, Zachman K, Crane M, Jezova D, Rovensky J, Dimitrov MA, Gold PW, Bonini S, Fleisher T, Chrousos GP, Wilder RL: Low- versus high-baseline epinephrine output shapes opposite innate cytokine profiles: presence of Lewis- and Fischer-like neurohormonal immune phenotypes in humans? J Immunol 2008;181:1737–1745.

42 Theoharides TC, Singh LK, Boucher W, Pang X, Letourneau R, Webster E, Chrousos GP: Corticotropin-releasing hormone induces skin mast cell degranulation and increased vascular permeability, a possible explanation for its proinflammatory effects. Endocrinology 1998;139:403–413.
43 Theoharides TC, Spanos C, Pang X, Alferes L, Ligris K, Letourneau R, Rozniecki JJ, Webster E, Chrousos GP: Stress-induced intracranial mast cell degranulation: a corticotropin-releasing hormone-mediated effect. Endocrinology 1995;136:5745–5750.
44 Burguera B, Muruais C, Penalva A, Dieguez C, Casanueva FF: Dual and selective actions of glucocorticoids upon basal and stimulated growth hormone release in man. Neuroendocrinology 1990;51:51–58.
45 Magiakou MA, Mastorakos G, Gomez MT, Rose SR, Chrousos GP: Suppressed spontaneous and stimulated growth hormone secretion in patients with Cushing's disease before and after surgical cure. J Clin Endocrinol Metab 1994;78:131–137.
46 Bamberger CM, Schulte HM, Chrousos GP: Molecular determinants of glucocorticoid receptor function and tissue sensitivity to glucocorticoids. Endocr Rev 1996;17:245–261.
47 Magiakou MA, Mastorakos G, Chrousos GP: Final stature in patients with endogenous Cushing's syndrome. J Clin Endocrinol Metab 1994;79:1082–1085.
48 Skuse D, Albanese A, Stanhope R, Gilmour J, Voss L: A new stress-related syndrome of growth failure and hyperphagia in children, associated with reversibility of growth hormone insufficiency. Lancet 1996;348:353–358.
49 Albanese A, Hamill G, Jones J, Skuse D, Matthews DR, Stanhope R: Reversibility of physiological growth hormone secretion in children with psychosocial dwarfism. Clin Endocrinol (Oxf) 1994;40:687–692.
50 Benker G, Raida M, Olbricht T, Wagner R, Reinhardt W, Reinwein D: TSH secretion in Cushing's syndrome: relation to glucocorticoid excess, diabetes, goitre and the 'sick euthyroid syndrome'. Clin Endocrinol (Oxf) 1990;33:777–786.
51 Whirledge S, Cidlowski JA: A role for glucocorticoids in stress-impaired reproduction: beyond the hypothalamus and pituitary. Endocrinology 2013;154:4450–4468.
52 Rivier C, Rivier J, Vale W: Stress-induced inhibition of reproductive functions: role of endogenous corticotropin-releasing factor. Science 1986;231:607–609.
53 Vamvakopoulos NC, Chrousos GP: Hormonal regulation of human corticotropin-releasing hormone gene expression: implications for the stress response and immune/inflammatory reaction. Endocr Rev 1994;15:409–420.
54 Chrousos GP, Torpy DJ, Gold PW: Interactions between the hypothalamic-pituitary-adrenal axis and the female reproductive system: clinical implications. Ann Intern Med 1998;129:229–240.
55 MacAdams MR, White RH, Chipps BE: Reduction of serum testosterone levels during chronic glucocorticoid therapy. Ann Intern Med 1986;104:648–651.
56 Luger A, Deuster PA, Kyle SB, Gallucci WT, Montgomery LC, Gold PW, Loriaux DL, Chrousos GP: Acute hypothalamic-pituitary-adrenal responses to the stress of treadmill exercise: physiologic adaptations to physical training. N Engl J Med 1987;316:1309–1315.
57 MacConnie SE, Barkan A, Lampman RM, Schork MA, Beitins IZ: Decreased hypothalamic gonadotropin-releasing hormone secretion in male marathon runners. N Engl J Med 1986;315:411–417.
58 Chrousos GP: The role of stress and the hypothalamic-pituitary-adrenal axis in the pathogenesis of the metabolic syndrome: neuroendocrine and target tissue-related causes. Int J Obes (London) 2000;24:s50f–s55f.
59 Chrousos GP, Tsigos C: Stress, obesity, and metabolic syndrome. Ann NY Acad Sci 2006;1083:xi–xiii.
60 Gold PW, Goodwin F, Chrousos GP: Clinical and biochemical manifestations of depression: relationship to the neurobiology of stress (part I). N Engl J Med 1988;319:348–353.
61 Gold PW, Goodwin F, Chrousos GP: Clinical and biochemical manifestations of depression: relationship to the neurobiology of stress (part II). N Engl J Med 1988;319:413–420.
62 Gold PW, Chrousos GP: Organization of the stress system and its dysregulation in melancholic and atypical depression: high vs. low CRH/NE states. Mol Psychiatry 2002;7:254–275.
63 Chrousos G: The glucocorticoid receptor gene, longevity, and the highly prevalent complex disorders of Western societies. Am J Med 2004;117:204–207.
64 Murgatroyd C, Wu Y, Bockmühl Y, Spengler D: Genes learn from stress: how infantile trauma programs us for depression. Epigenetics 2010;5:194–199.
65 Meaney MJ, Aitken DH, Bodnoff SR, Iny LJ, Tatarewicz JE, Sapolsky RM: Early postnatal handling alters glucocorticoid receptor concentrations in selected brain regions. Behav Neurosci 1985;99:765–770.
66 Meaney MJ, Aitken DH, Sapolsky RM: Thyroid hormones influence the development of hippocampal glucocorticoid receptors in the rat: a mechanism for the effects of postnatal handling on the development of the adrenocortical stress response. Neuroendocrinology 1987;45:278–283.
67 Mitchell JB, Iny LJ, Meaney MJ: The role of serotonin in the development and environmental regulation of type II corticosteroid receptor binding in rat hippocampus. Brain Res Dev Brain Res 1990;55:231–235.
68 Champagne FA: Early environments, glucocorticoid receptors, and behavioral epigenetics. Behav Neurosci 2013;127:628–636.
69 Liu D, Diorio J, Tannenbaum B, Caldji C, Francis D, Freedman A, Sharma S, Pearson D, Plotsky PM, Meaney MJ: Maternal care, hippocampal glucocorticoid receptors, and hypothalamic-pituitary-adrenal responses to stress. Science 1997;277:1659–1662.
70 Hellstrom IC, Dhir SK, Diorio JC, Meaney MJ: Maternal licking regulates hippocampal glucocorticoid receptor transcription through a thyroid hormone-serotonin-NGFI-A signalling cascade. Philos Trans R Soc Lond B Biol Sci 2012;367:2495–2510.
71 Weaver IC, Cervoni N, Champagne FA, D'Alessio AC, Sharma S, Seckl JR, Dymov S, Szyf M, Meaney MJ: Epigenetic programming by maternal behavior. Nature Neuroscience 2004;7:847–854.
72 McGowan PO, Sasaki A, D'Alessio AC, Dymov S, Labonté B, Szyf M, Turecki G, Meaney MJ: Epigenetic regulation of the glucocorticoid receptor in human brain associates with childhood abuse. Nat Neurosci 2009;12:342–348.
73 Stankiewicz AM, Swiergiel AH, Lisowski P: Epigenetics of stress adaptations in the brain. Brain Res Bull 2013;98:76–92.
74 Weaver IC, Champagne FA, Brown SE, Dymov S, Sharma S, Meaney MJ, Szyf M: Reversal of maternal programming of stress responses in adult offspring through methyl supplementation: altering epigenetic marking later in life. J Neurosci 2005;25:11045–11054.
75 Meaney MJ: Nature, nurture, and the disunity of knowledge. Ann NY Acad Sci 2001;935:50–61.

NeuroImmunoModulation

Neuroimmunomodulation 2015;22:20–32
DOI: 10.1159/000362724

Published online: September 12, 2014

One Hormone, Two Actions: Anti- and Pro-Inflammatory Effects of Glucocorticoids

Diana Cruz-Topete John A. Cidlowski

Laboratory of Signal Transduction, National Institute of Environmental Health Sciences (NIEHS), National Institutes of Health, Department of Health and Human Services, Research Triangle Park, N.C., USA

Key Words

Glucocorticoids · Stress hormones · Glucocorticoid receptor · Inflammation · Immunity · Pro-inflammatory and anti-inflammatory

Abstract

Glucocorticoids are essential steroid hormones secreted from the adrenal gland in response to stress. Since their discovery in the 1940s, glucocorticoids have been widely prescribed to treat inflammatory disorders and hematological cancers. In the traditional view, glucocorticoids are regarded as anti-inflammatory molecules; however, emerging evidence suggests that glucocorticoid actions are more complex than previously anticipated. The anti-inflammatory activity of glucocorticoids is attributed to the repression of pro-inflammatory genes through signal transduction by their steroid receptor, the glucocorticoid receptor (GR). The mechanisms modulating the pro-inflammatory effects of glucocorticoids are not well understood. In this review, we discuss recent findings that provide insights into the mechanism by which GR signaling can play a dual role in the regulation of the immune response. We hypothesize that these apparently opposite processes are working together to prepare the immune system to respond to a stressor (pro-inflammatory effects) and subsequently restore homeostasis (anti-inflammatory effects). Finally, we propose that determining the mechanisms which underlie the tissue-specific effects of glucocorticoids will provide an excellent tool to develop more efficient and selective glucocorticoid therapies.

Glucocorticoids and the Stress Response

Glucocorticoids are steroid hormones synthesized and secreted by the adrenal gland in response to stress [1]. Upon exposure to stress, the hypothalamus is stimulated to release corticotrophin-releasing hormone, which then acts on the anterior pituitary gland to stimulate the synthesis of adrenocorticotropic hormone (ACTH). ACTH then acts on the adrenal cortex to induce the secretion of glucocorticoids [2]. Once in circulation, glucocorticoids exert a variety of tissue-specific effects (fig. 1) [2–5]. Therefore, glucocorticoid imbalances can result in pathological conditions such as the severe cardiovascular, metabolic and immunological complications observed in Cushing's syndrome (glucocorticoid excess) and Addison's disease (glucocorticoid deficiency).

KARGER

E-Mail karger@karger.com
www.karger.com/nim

1021–7401/14/0222–0020$39.50/0

Dr. John A. Cidlowski
Laboratory of Signal Transduction
National Institute of Environmental Health Sciences
Research Triangle Park, NC 27709 (USA)
E-Mail cidlows1@niehs.nih.gov

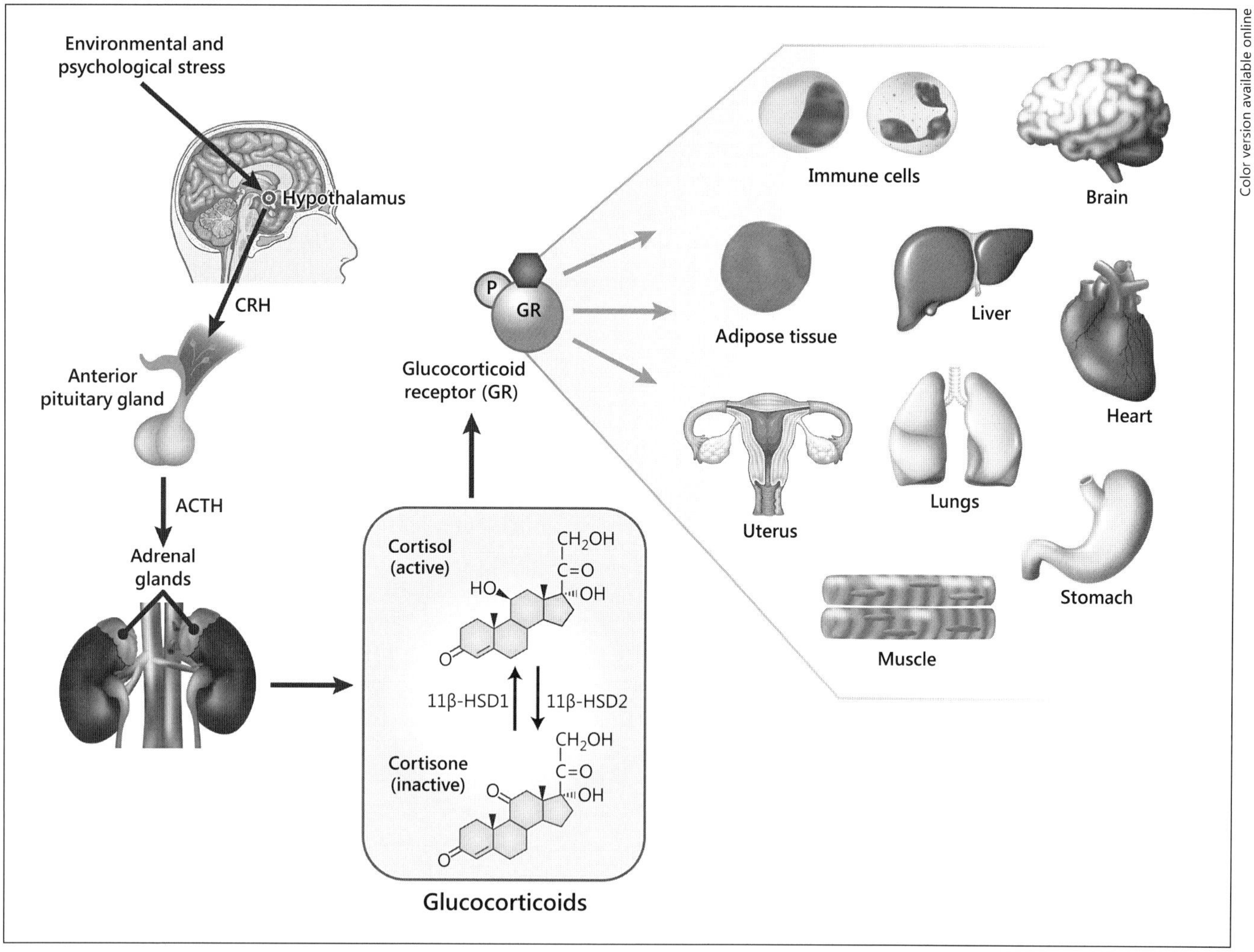

Fig. 1. Regulation of glucocorticoid secretion in response to stress by the hypothalamic-pituitary-adrenal axis. Upon exposure to environmental or psychological stress the hypothalamus is stimulated to release corticotropin-releasing hormone (CRH). CRH then stimulates the anterior pituitary gland to secrete ACTH. In turn, ACTH targets the cortex of the adrenal glands to release cortisol into the bloodstream. Once in circulation, cortisol can be converted to the inactive form, cortisone, by 11β-hydroxysteroid dehydrogenase type 2. Conversely, 11β-hydroxysteroid dehydrogenase type 1 converts cortisone to cortisol. Glucocorticoids exert their effects by binding to their receptor, the GR. GR is expressed in virtually all cell types and tissues. Thus, GR signaling plays an important role in the modulation of a large number of biological functions in immune cells and in several organs and tissues, including the brain, liver, heart, lungs, adipose tissue, reproductive system, stomach and muscle.

Glucocorticoid therapy was first introduced by Dr. Philip Hench in the 1940s for the treatment of rheumatoid arthritis [6]. Since then, glucocorticoids have commonly been prescribed to treat inflammatory disorders, including asthma, allergic rhinitis, ulcerative colitis, and several other dermatological, ophthalmic, neurological and autoimmune diseases [7, 8]. Despite their therapeutic benefits, glucocorticoid use, in traditional high doses >5 mg/day, is associated with severe side effects, including diabetes, hypertension, glaucoma, muscle atrophy and growth retardation [7, 9]. However, the magnitude of the positive or negative effects of glucocorticoids will depend on the dose, duration of the treatment, glucocorticoid receptor (GR) levels, and cell- and tissue-specific glucocorticoid signal transduction [10–12].

Long-term treatment with glucocorticoids can also be associated with glucocorticoid resistance, which results in the inability of glucocorticoids to exert their effects on target tissues, limiting the efficacy of the therapy [13]. Therefore, understanding how glucocorticoids exert their actions in a dose- and tissue-specific manner should help to develop novel therapies using these agents that may decrease their undesired effects. This review examines evidence that emphasizes the pro- and anti-inflammatory actions of glucocorticoids on the immune system. These apparently opposite effects appear to work together as a defense mechanism to 'prepare' the immune system to respond to a stressor, and subsequently to shut down the immune response to restore homeostasis [14].

Molecular Mechanisms of Glucocorticoids

GR Structure

Glucocorticoids exert their actions by binding to their receptor, the GR, a ligand-induced transcription factor and member of the nuclear receptor superfamily [15]. GR is expressed in virtually all cell types and tissues [1, 3, 8]. In terms of the structure, GR is composed of 3 major functional domains: the N-terminal domain (NTD); the central DNA-binding domain (DBD); the C-terminal ligand-binding domain (LBD), as well as a hinge region (region linking the DBD and LBD; fig. 2a) [2, 14]. Each domain comprises a specific function; for example, the NTD has a transcriptional activation function (AF)-1 domain which contains the majority of the residues subject to post-translational modifications (PTMs). The NTD is important for the recruitment of the basal transcriptional machinery. The DBD consists of two zinc fingers implicated in DNA binding, nuclear translocation and GR dimerization [2]. The LBD also contains an AF-2 domain which interacts with co-regulators in a ligand-dependent manner [14, 16–18].

GR Genomic and Non-Genomic Effects

Under basal conditions, GR resides primarily in the cytoplasm in a complex with chaperone proteins hsp90, hsp70 and p23, and immunophilins FKBP51 and FKBP52, where it is largely considered to be functionless [2, 5]. Upon hormone binding, GR translocates into the nucleus to enhance or repress the transcription of target genes by several mechanisms: (1) direct binding to specific *cis*-acting DNA sequences (glucocorticoid-responsive elements; GREs); (2) tethering itself to other transcription factors, and/or (3) through direct binding to DNA and interacting with neighboring transcription factors, which is known as composite regulation (fig. 2b) [2].

The GRE consensus sequence is GAGAACAnnnT-GTTCT, an imperfect palindrome containing two hexameric half sites separated by three base pairs [18–20]. GR binding to GREs typically leads to transactivation, where glucocorticoids induce target genes. However, recent studies have shown that GR occupancy of a GRE can also lead to gene repression, in a process known as 'transrepression' (fig. 2b) [21]. GR can also repress genes by tethering itself to other transcription factors. For example, GR can physically interact with nuclear factor-κB (NF-κB) and activator protein-1 (AP-1), which represses their capacity to induce the transcription of pro-inflammatory genes (fig. 2b) [22, 23]. GR is also known to bind to inverted palindromic sequences denominated as negative GREs (nGREs). The consensus sequence of these *cis*-acting negative response elements is CTCC(n)0–2GGAGA [24]. Studies have shown that GR recruitment to nGREs promotes the assembly of a corepressor complex and the recruitment of histone deacetylases, which direct glucocorticoid-dependent repression of specific genes [25] (fig. 2b).

GR has also been proposed to exert 'rapid' non-genomic actions by directly modulating signal transduction pathways [2]. This process occurs via membrane-bound GR or cytosolic GR interactions with kinases, such as the ERKs (extracellular signal-regulated kinases), the JNKs (c-Jun NH2-terminal kinases), the p38s (p38 isoforms), and ERK5 [26] (fig. 2b). To date, the detailed mechanism and biological implications of non-genomic effects of GR have not been fully elucidated; human studies suggest that this response might have important physiological effects on the cardiovascular and immune system [26, 27]. Non-genomic effects of glucocorticoids are extensively discussed in a recent publication by Ayroldi et al. [26].

GR Isoforms

In addition to the genomic and non-genomic actions of glucocorticoids, GR signaling is also dependent on the existence of multiple receptor isoforms and PTMs [2, 4]. GR is transcribed from a single gene, *NR3C1*. However, alternative splicing of this gene generates GRα and GRβ isoforms, which differ in their C-terminal domain [28]. Both isoforms are associated with distinct responses to glucocorticoids [29]. The existence of different isoforms explains in part how a 'single' receptor can exert a plethora of pharmacological and cellular responses. Human GRα, the classical GR protein, exerts most of the biological actions of glucocorticoids [29]. Furthermore, GRα expression is higher than GRβ in tissues [30]. In general, GRβ presents several distinct properties: it is located pri-

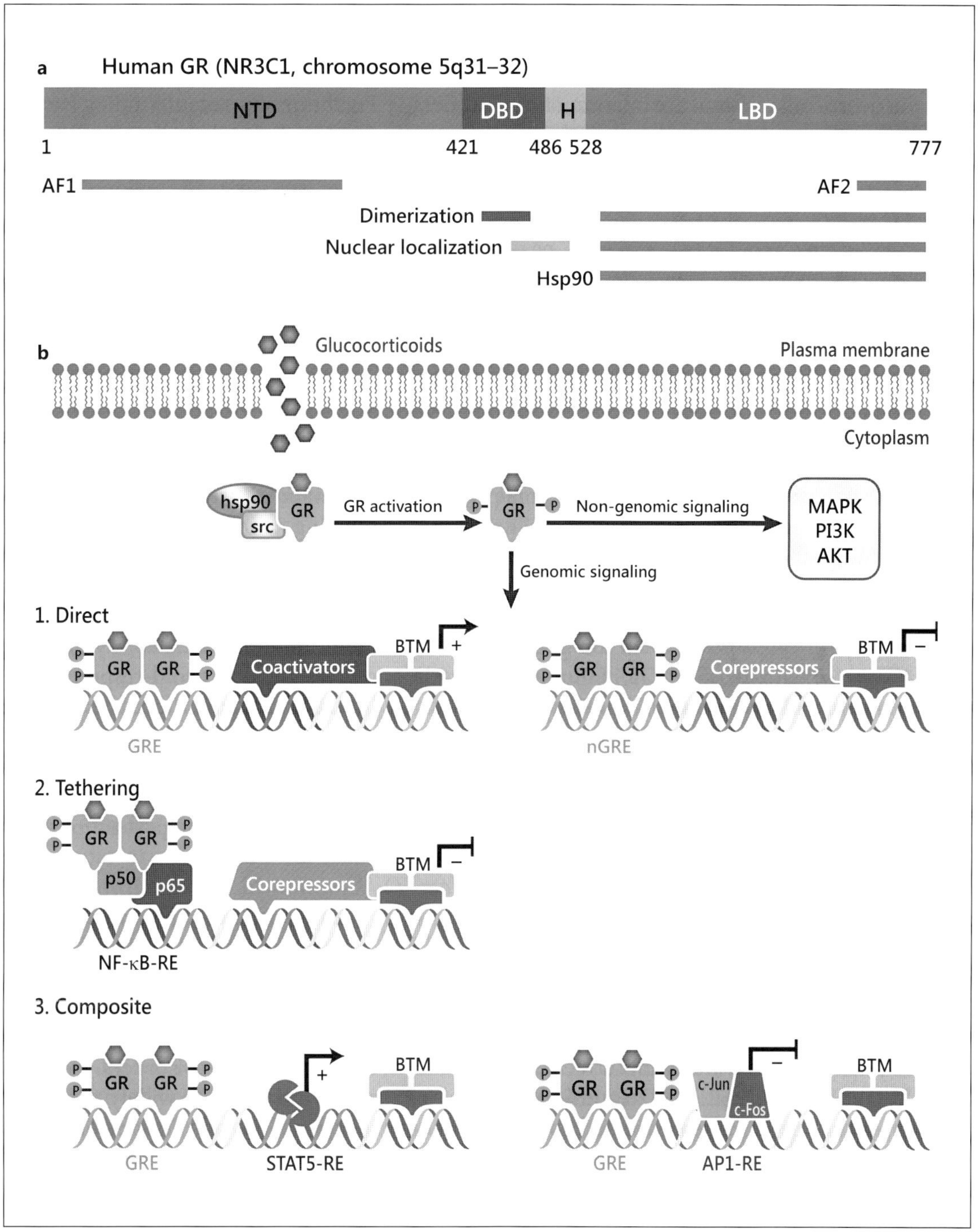

Fig. 2. Schematic representation of the GR structure and signaling pathways. **a** GR domains and regions involved in transactivation (AF1 and AF2), dimerization, nuclear localization and Hsp90 binding. H = Hinge region. **b** GR can signal in a non-genomic manner by modulating the activity of several kinases, including MAPK, phosphoinositide 3-kinase (PI3K) and AKT. GR regulates gene expression by three mechanisms: (1) direct – activated GR binds to GREs or nGREs on the promoter or sequence of target genes; (2) tethering – GR tethers itself to other DNA-bound transcription factors; (3) composite – GR binds directly to a GRE and interacts with neighboring DNA-bound transcription factors. BTM = Basal transcription machinery; STAT = signal transducer and activator of transcription.

lin (TTP) [66]. TTP plays an important role in the resolution phase of the inflammatory response by destabilizing the mRNA of many pro-inflammatory cytokines and targeting them for degradation [67], and dexamethasone (a synthetic glucocorticoid) treatment of A549 lung epithelial cells induces TTP gene expression [66]. These studies provide evidence that glucocorticoids can repress the inflammatory process indirectly via the induction of anti-inflammatory molecules. In summary, glucocorticoids can modulate inflammation directly at the transcriptional level by repressing the gene expression of pro-inflammatory molecules, or through post-transcriptional mechanisms via interactions with anti-inflammatory proteins.

Pro-Inflammatory Effects of Glucocorticoids

Glucocorticoid secretion in response to stress has been assumed mainly to be anti-inflammatory, as discussed above. However, studies suggest that the type of exposure to glucocorticoids and the basal state of the immune system are important factors influencing the effects of glucocorticoids [47, 48, 50–52, 68]. For example, while chronic exposure to glucocorticoids seems to be immunosuppressive, acute exposure enhances the peripheral immune response [48]. The mechanisms by which the same hormone directs opposite responses are not well understood.

Genome-wide microarray studies of human mononuclear cells suggest that glucocorticoids can induce the expression of several innate immune-related genes, including several members of the Toll-like receptor (TLR) family [69, 70]. However, in the same cells, glucocorticoids have an inhibitory effect on the expression of pro-inflammatory genes of the adaptive immune response [70]. These findings are interesting because it is generally accepted that glucocorticoids suppress TLRs – the activation of which is a hallmark feature of inflammation – through the induction of MKP-1 or glucocorticoid-induced leucine zipper, or via repression of AP-1 and NF-κB [69].

GR signaling interplays with TLR signaling pathways through several mechanisms [14]. For the purpose of this review, we will discuss briefly the mechanisms that enhance the activity of TLRs (fig. 5a). Several studies have reported that glucocorticoids induce the expression of TLR2 and TLR4 in lung epithelial cells [69, 71, 72]. Interestingly, glucocorticoids have also been shown to increase *Haemophilus influenzae*-induced expression of TLR2 mRNA and protein levels via negative cross-talk with p38 MAPK [73]. A study by Hermoso et al. [72] showed that dexamethasone enhances TNF-α induction of TLR2 via the activation of GR.

TNF-α and dexamethasone drive the binding of NF-κB and STAT to their respective consensus sequences in the TLR2 promoter, leading to TLR2 induction. Furthermore, chromatin immunoprecipitation (ChIP) assays showed that GR is recruited to the TLR2 proximal promoter region in response to dexamethasone, which perhaps contributes to GR-TNF-α effects on TLR2 expression [72]. Although these results appear paradoxical, studies in TLR2 knockout mice have shown that TLR2 deficiency is associated with reduced corticosterone levels, morphological alterations in adrenocortical tissue and impairments in the activation of the inflammatory response following LPS administration [74]. Therefore, these results support the existence of positive feedback between glucocorticoid secretion and the activation of the TLR signaling pathway.

Interestingly, genome-wide microarray studies in A549 cells treated with dexamethasone and TNF-α showed that more than 800 genes were co-regulated significantly by dexamethasone and TNF-α, including the acute-phase protein SerpinA3 secreted into circulation during acute and chronic inflammation [75]. In vitro and in vivo co-administration of glucocorticoids and TNF-α resulted in synergetic increases of SerpinA3 mRNA and protein levels. In addition, ChIP assays indicate that GR binding at the SerpinA3 transcription start site is more robust when cells are co-treated with dexamethasone and TNF-α [75]. These data revealed a novel signaling pathway by which glucocorticoids exert pro-inflammatory actions via interactions with inflammatory cytokines. These results provide a potential explanation for some of the negative side effects of long-term glucocorticoid treatment.

Genome-wide ChIP-chip assays showed that treatment of AtT-20 (pituitary adenoma cell line) cells with leukemia inhibitory factor (LIF), a member of the IL-6 family, and/or dexamethasone potentiates STAT3 and GR recruitment to many STAT3 target genes [76]. LIF signaling on its own was found to modulate a very limited gene subset while dexamethasone co-administrated with LIF leads to a significant upregulation in the expression of genes involved in the cellular defense response, including genes involved in the innate immune response and in the hepatic acute-phase response [76]. Interestingly, similar results were observed in vivo in response to LIF-dexamethasone co-treatment [76]. Therefore, glucocorticoids can work synergistically with pro-inflammatory media-

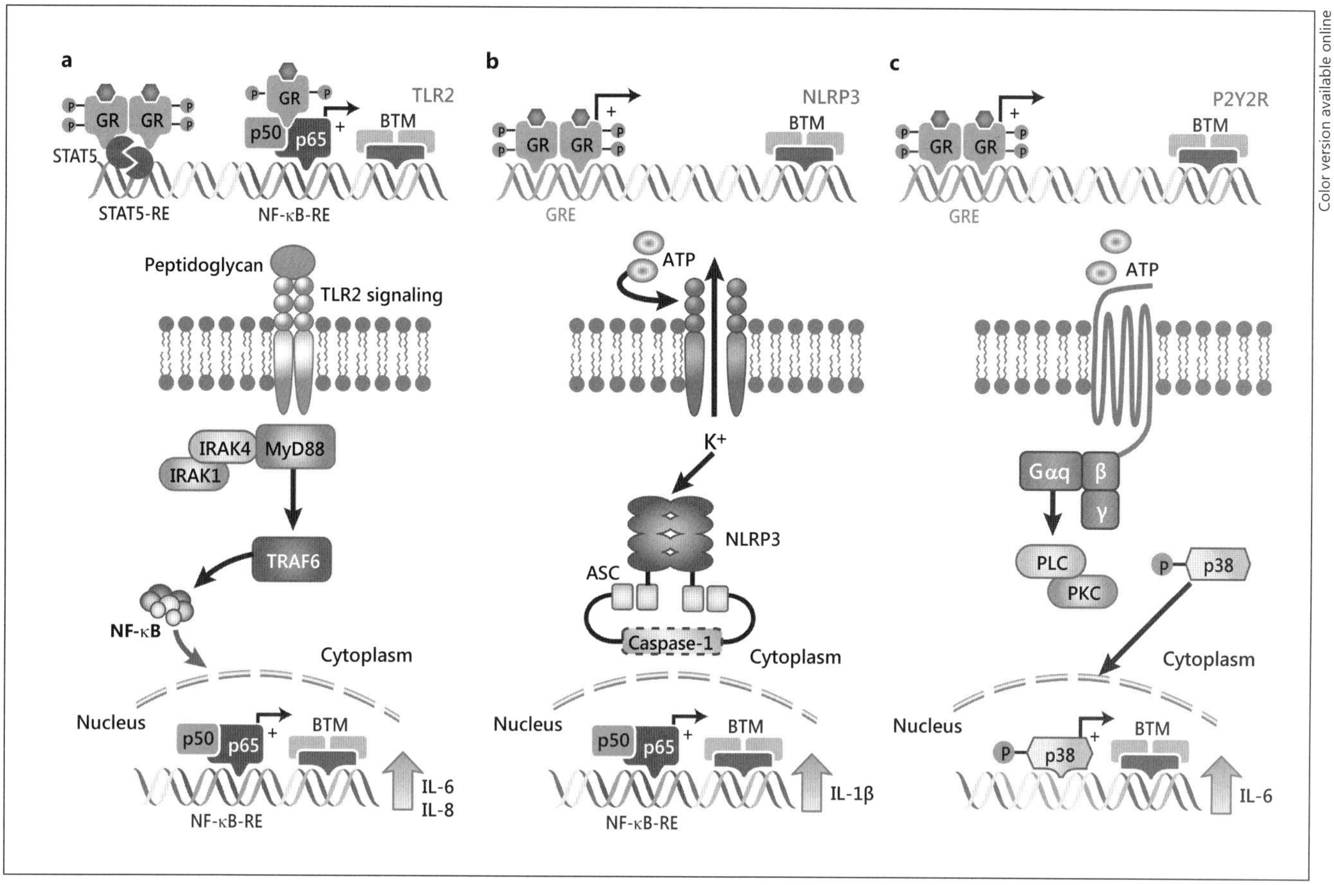

Fig. 5. Glucocorticoid-mediated modulation of pro-inflammatory pathways. **a** GR can drive the expression of TLR2 by interacting with STAT5 and NF-κB. TLR2 recognizes the bacterial cell wall component peptidoglycan. Upon stimulation, MYD88 binds to the cytoplasmic portion of TLR2. This event leads to recruitment and activation of IRAK1, IRAK4 and TRAF6, ultimately leading to the downstream signaling activation of pro-inflammatory transcription factors which drives the expression of inflammatory cytokines, including IL-6 and IL-8. **b**, **c** Glucocorticoids regulate the expression of NLRP3 and P2Y2R by mechanisms that are not well understood. NLRP3 regulates the immune system response to injury or pathogens by sensitizing macrophages to extracellular ATP (danger signal) and inducing the synthesis of IL-1β. P2Y2R is a G-protein-coupled receptor that is activated in response to ATP, which stimulates the activation of PLC (phospholipase C) and PKC (protein kinase C), and the subsequent downstream signaling. Glucocorticoids can upregulate the expression of P2Y2R by enhancing the ATP-dependent activation of p38, which leads to the expression of the pro-inflammatory cytokine IL-6.

tors to reinforce the defense mechanisms to ensure clearance and removal of pathogens [14, 76].

Glucocorticoids have also been shown to induce the expression of the NOD-like receptor family, pyrin domain containing 3 gene (NLRP3), a central component of the inflammasome, in both cultured and primary macrophages (fig. 5b) [77]. Glucocorticoid induction of NLRP3 sensitized macrophages to extracellular ATP, which resulted in the secretion of pro-inflammatory cytokines, IL-1β, TNF-α and IL-6 [77]. In addition, glucocorticoids have been reported to induce the expression of the purinergic receptor P2Y2R (fig. 5c). Activation of P2Y2R enhances IL-6 secretion by endothelial cells in response to ATP [78]. Thus, glucocorticoid-mediated activation of TLR2, NLRP3, P2Y2R and potentiation of TNF-α- and LIF-regulated pro-inflammatory genes provide a potential mechanism by which these hormones exert pro-inflammatory actions in response to stress [14].

Concluding Remarks

The discovery that glucocorticoids, the most widely prescribed drugs for the treatment of inflammatory disorders, can exert both pro-and anti-inflammatory actions suggests that the effects of glucocorticoids are more complex than previously recognized. The mechanism(s) by which the same protein can regulate these two opposing processes is only beginning to be understood.

The positive regulation of components of the innate immune response suggests that glucocorticoids prepare the immune system for a quick and efficient response to pathogens [14]. Thus, glucocorticoid-mediated initial pro-inflammatory activity is perhaps required for a functional immune system. Studies on T cell receptor-deficient mice have shown that GR expression is essential for survival during polyclonal T cell activation. GR modulates the activation of both Th1 and Th2 cells, and limits the severity of the inflammatory process by regulating T cell expression of pro-inflammatory molecules [79]. In humans, glucocorticoid deficiency is commonly associated with a defective immune response and recurrent infections [80]. In addition, studies on adrenalectomized rats showed that complete removal of glucocorticoids leads to an increase in susceptibility to LPS-induced inflammation [81]. These findings suggest that glucocorticoids play an important role in priming the immune system to respond to injury, and controlling the release of inflammatory molecules to prevent an overreaction.

In summary, the nature of the response to glucocorticoids relies on several factors, including the duration of the stimulus (acute or chronic) and the physiological state of the immune system. In pathological situations, glucocorticoids may function as anti-inflammatory molecules to control the process. In contrast, under normal physiological conditions, glucocorticoids may play a pro-inflammatory role.

Future studies are needed to characterize the tissue-specific effects of the pro- and anti-inflammatory roles of GR signaling. Understanding of the physiological effects of glucocorticoids should enable us to decipher the mechanisms governing GR actions, and ultimately to develop therapeutic strategies to take advantage of the capacity of GR to elicit pro-and anti-inflammatory effects.

Acknowledgments

We would like to apologize to those colleagues whose work we were unable to cite owing to space limitations. We would like to thank these individuals for all their work that has significantly contributed to our understanding of GR molecular actions. We also would like to thank Dr. Mahita Kadmiel, Dr. Sivapriya Ramamoorthy, Dr. Shannon Whirledge and Alyson Scoltock for their helpful input. Finally, we would like to acknowledge NIEHS arts and photography for their assistance. This work was supported by the NIEHS Intramural Research Program of the National Institutes of Health.

References

1 Sapolsky RM, Romero LM, Munck AU: How do glucocorticoids influence stress responses? Integrating permissive, suppressive, stimulatory, and preparative actions. Endocr Rev 2000;21:55–89.
2 Oakley RH, Cidlowski JA: The biology of the glucocorticoid receptor: new signaling mechanisms in health and disease. J Allergy Clin Immunol 2013;132:1033–1044.
3 Kadmiel M, Cidlowski JA: Glucocorticoid receptor signaling in health and disease. Trends Pharmacol Sci 2013;34:518–530.
4 Zhou J, Cidlowski JA: The human glucocorticoid receptor: one gene, multiple proteins and diverse responses. Steroids 2005;70:407–417.
5 Vandevyver S, Dejager L, Tuckermann J, Libert C: New insights into the anti-inflammatory mechanisms of glucocorticoids: an emerging role for glucocorticoid-receptor-mediated transactivation. Endocrinology 2013;154:993–1007.
6 Clark AR, Belvisi MG: Maps and legends: the quest for dissociated ligands of the glucocorticoid receptor. Pharmacol Ther 2012;134: 54–67.
7 Rhen T, Cidlowski JA: Antiinflammatory action of glucocorticoids – new mechanisms for old drugs. N Engl J Med 2005;353:1711–1723.
8 Nussinovitch U, de Carvalho JF, Pereira RM, Shoenfeld Y: Glucocorticoids and the cardiovascular system: state of the art. Curr Pharm Des 2010;16:3574–3585.
9 Miner JN, Hong MH, Negro-Vilar A: New and improved glucocorticoid receptor ligands. Expert Opin Investig Drugs 2005;14: 1527–1545.
10 Vanderbilt JN, Miesfeld R, Maler BA, Yamamoto KR: Intracellular receptor concentration limits glucocorticoid-dependent enhancer activity. Mol Endocrinol 1987;1:68–74.
11 Danielsen M, Stallcup MR: Down-regulation of glucocorticoid receptors in mouse lymphoma cell variants. Mol Cell Biol 1984;4:449–453.
12 Silva CM, Lu H, Weber MJ, Thorner MO: Differential tyrosine phosphorylation of JAK1, JAK2, and STAT1 by growth hormone and interferon-gamma in IM-9 cells. J Biol Chem 1994;269:27532–27539.
13 Barnes PJ, Adcock IM: Glucocorticoid resistance in inflammatory diseases. Lancet 2009; 373:1905–1917.
14 Busillo JM, Cidlowski JA: The five Rs of glucocorticoid action during inflammation: ready, reinforce, repress, resolve, and restore. Trends Endocrinol Metab 2013;24:109–119.
15 Whitfield GK, Jurutka PW, Haussler CA, Haussler MR: Steroid hormone receptors: evolution, ligands, and molecular basis of biologic function. J Cell Biochem 1999;suppl 32–33:110–122.
16 Hollenberg SM, Weinberger C, Ong ES, Cerelli G, Oro A, Lebo R, Thompson EB, Rosenfeld MG, Evans RM: Primary structure and expression of a functional human glucocorticoid receptor cDNA. Nature 1985;318:635–641.
17 Nicolaides NC, Galata Z, Kino T, Chrousos GP, Charmandari E: The human glucocorticoid receptor: molecular basis of biologic function. Steroids 2010;75:1–12.
18 Beck IM, De Bosscher K, Haegeman G: Glucocorticoid receptor mutants: man-made tools for functional research. Trends Endocrinol Metab 2011;22:295–310.
19 Beato M: Gene regulation by steroid hormones. Cell 1989;56:335–344.

20 Freedman LP: Anatomy of the steroid receptor zinc finger region. Endocr Rev 1992;13: 129–145.
21 Uhlenhaut NH, Barish GD, Yu RT, Downes M, Karunasiri M, Liddle C, Schwalie P, Hubner N, Evans RM: Insights into negative regulation by the glucocorticoid receptor from genome-wide profiling of inflammatory cistromes. Mol Cell 2013;49:158–171.
22 De Bosscher K, Vanden Berghe W, Haegeman G: Mechanisms of anti-inflammatory action and of immunosuppression by glucocorticoids: negative interference of activated glucocorticoid receptor with transcription factors. J Neuroimmunol 2000;109:16–22.
23 De Bosscher K, Vanden Berghe W, Vermeulen L, Plaisance S, Boone E, Haegeman G: Glucocorticoids repress NF-κB-driven genes by disturbing the interaction of p65 with the basal transcription machinery, irrespective of coactivator levels in the cell. Proc Natl Acad Sci USA 2000;97:3919–3924.
24 So AY, Chaivorapol C, Bolton EC, Li H, Yamamoto KR: Determinants of cell and gene-specific transcriptional regulation by the glucocorticoid receptor. PLoS Genet 2007;3:e94.
25 Surjit M, Ganti KP, Mukherji A, Ye T, Hua G, Metzger D, Li M, Chambon P: Widespread negative response elements mediate direct repression by agonist-liganded glucocorticoid receptor. Cell 2011;145:224–241.
26 Ayroldi E, Cannarile L, Migliorati G, Nocentini G, Delfino DV, Riccardi C: Mechanisms of the anti-inflammatory effects of glucocorticoids: genomic and nongenomic interference with MAPK signaling pathways. Faseb J 2012;26:4805–4820.
27 Lee SR, Kim HK, Youm JB, Dizon LA, Song IS, Jeong SH, Seo DY, Ko KS, Rhee BD, Kim N, et al: Non-genomic effect of glucocorticoids on cardiovascular system. Pflügers Arch 2012;464:549–559.
28 Yudt MR, Cidlowski JA: Molecular identification and characterization of A and B forms of the glucocorticoid receptor. Mol Endocrinol 2001;15:1093–1103.
29 Gross KL, Cidlowski JA: Tissue-specific glucocorticoid action: a family affair. Trends Endocrinol Metab 2008;19:331–339.
30 Oakley RH, Sar M, Cidlowski JA: The human glucocorticoid receptor β isoform. Expression, biochemical properties, and putative function. J Biol Chem 1996;271:9550–9559.
31 Oakley RH, Cidlowski JA: Cellular processing of the glucocorticoid receptor gene and protein: new mechanisms for generating tissue-specific actions of glucocorticoids. J Biol Chem 2011;286:3177–3184.
32 Bamberger CM, Bamberger AM, de Castro M, Chrousos GP: Glucocorticoid receptor beta, a potential endogenous inhibitor of glucocorticoid action in humans. J Clin Invest 1995;95: 2435–2441.
33 Kino T, Su YA, Chrousos GP: Human glucocorticoid receptor isoform beta: recent understanding of its potential implications in physiology and pathophysiology. Cell Mol Life Sci 2009;66:3435–3448.
34 Lewis-Tuffin LJ, Cidlowski JA: The physiology of human glucocorticoid receptor beta (hGRβ) and glucocorticoid resistance. Ann NY Acad Sci 2006;1069:1–9.
35 Kino T, Manoli I, Kelkar S, Wang Y, Su YA, Chrousos GP: Glucocorticoid receptor (GR) β has intrinsic, GRα-independent transcriptional activity. Biochem Biophys Res Commun 2009;381:671–675.
36 Avenant C, Ronacher K, Stubsrud E, Louw A, Hapgood JP: Role of ligand-dependent GR phosphorylation and half-life in determination of ligand-specific transcriptional activity. Mol Cell Endocrinol 2010;327:72–88.
37 Wang Z, Frederick J, Garabedian MJ: Deciphering the phosphorylation 'code' of the glucocorticoid receptor in vivo. J Biol Chem 2002;277:26573–26580.
38 Webster JC, Jewell CM, Bodwell JE, Munck A, Sar M, Cidlowski JA: Mouse glucocorticoid receptor phosphorylation status influences multiple functions of the receptor protein. J Biol Chem 1997;272:9287–9293.
39 Miller AL, Webb MS, Copik AJ, Wang Y, Johnson BH, Kumar R, Thompson EB: p38 mitogen-activated protein kinase (MAPK) is a key mediator in glucocorticoid-induced apoptosis of lymphoid cells: correlation between p38 MAPK activation and site-specific phosphorylation of the human glucocorticoid receptor at serine 211. Mol Endocrinol 2005; 19:1569–1583.
40 Chen W, Dang T, Blind RD, Wang Z, Cavasotto CN, Hittelman AB, Rogatsky I, Logan SK, Garabedian MJ: Glucocorticoid receptor phosphorylation differentially affects target gene expression. Mol Endocrinol 2008;22: 1754–1766.
41 Galliher-Beckley AJ, Williams JG, Collins JB, Cidlowski JA: Glycogen synthase kinase 3β-mediated serine phosphorylation of the human glucocorticoid receptor redirects gene expression profiles. Mol Cell Biol 2008;28: 73097322.
42 Galliher-Beckley AJ, Williams JG, Cidlowski JA: Ligand-independent phosphorylation of the glucocorticoid receptor integrates cellular stress pathways with nuclear receptor signaling. Mol Cell Biol 2011;31:4663–4675.
43 Wallace AD, Cidlowski JA: Proteasome-mediated glucocorticoid receptor degradation restricts transcriptional signaling by glucocorticoids. J Biol Chem 2001;276:42714–42721.
44 Druker J, Liberman AC, Antunica-Noguerol M, Gerez J, Paez-Pereda M, Rein T, Iniguez-Lluhi JA, Holsboer F, Arzt E: RSUME enhances glucocorticoid receptor SUMOylation and transcriptional activity. Mol Cell Biol 2013; 33:2116–2127.
45 Ito K, Yamamura S, Essilfie-Quaye S, Cosio B, Ito M, Barnes PJ, Adcock IM: Histone deacetylase 2-mediated deacetylation of the glucocorticoid receptor enables NF-κB suppression. J Exp Med 2006;203:7–13.
46 Charmandari E, Chrousos GP, Lambrou GI, Pavlaki A, Koide H, Ng SS, Kino T: Peripheral CLOCK regulates target-tissue glucocorticoid receptor transcriptional activity in a circadian fashion in man. PLoS One 2011; 6:e25612.
47 Sorrells SF, Sapolsky RM: An inflammatory review of glucocorticoid actions in the CNS. Brain Behav Immun 2007;21:259–272.
48 Dhabhar FS: Stress-induced augmentation of immune function – the role of stress hormones, leukocyte trafficking, and cytokines. Brain Behav Immun 2002;16:785–798.
49 Dhabhar FS, McEwen BS: Enhancing versus suppressive effects of stress hormones on skin immune function. Proc Natl Acad Sci USA 1999;96:1059–1064.
50 Deinzer R, Granrath N, Stuhl H, Twork L, Idel H, Waschul B, Herforth A: Acute stress effects on local Il-1β responses to pathogens in a human in vivo model. Brain Behav Immun 2004; 18:458–467.
51 O'Connor KA, Johnson JD, Hansen MK, Wieseler Frank JL, Maksimova E, Watkins LR, Maier SF: Peripheral and central proinflammatory cytokine response to a severe acute stressor. Brain Res 2003;991:123–132.
52 Bowers SL, Bilbo SD, Dhabhar FS, Nelson RJ: Stressor-specific alterations in corticosterone and immune responses in mice. Brain Behav Immun 2008;22:105–113.
53 Akira S, Uematsu S, Takeuchi O: Pathogen recognition and innate immunity. Cell 2006; 124:783–801.
54 Pancer Z, Cooper MD: The evolution of adaptive immunity. Annu Rev Immunol 2006;24: 497–518.
55 Bhattacharyya S, Brown DE, Brewer JA, Vogt SK, Muglia LJ: Macrophage glucocorticoid receptors regulate Toll like receptor 4-mediated inflammatory responses by selective inhibition of p38 MAP kinase. Blood 2007;109: 4313–4319.
56 Tuckermann JP, Kleiman A, Moriggl R, Spanbroek R, Neumann A, Illing A, Clausen BE, Stride B, Forster I, Habenicht AJ, et al: Macrophages and neutrophils are the targets for immune suppression by glucocorticoids in contact allergy. J Clin Invest 2007;117:1381–1390.
57 Barnes PJ: How corticosteroids control inflammation: Quintiles Prize Lecture 2005. Br J Pharmacol 2006;148:245–254.
58 Hess J, Angel P, Schorpp-Kistner M: AP-1 subunits: quarrel and harmony among siblings. J Cell Sci 2004;117(pt 25):5965–5973.
59 Johnson GL, Lapadat R: Mitogen-activated protein kinase pathways mediated by ERK, JNK, and p38 protein kinases. Science 2002; 298:1911–1912.

60 Kumar A, Takada Y, Boriek AM, Aggarwal BB: Nuclear factor-κB: its role in health and disease. J Mol Med (Berl) 2004;82:434–448.
61 Liden J, Delaunay F, Rafter I, Gustafsson J, Okret S: A new function for the C-terminal zinc finger of the glucocorticoid receptor: repression of RelA transactivation. J Biol Chem 1997;272:21467–21472.
62 Reily MM, Pantoja C, Hu X, Chinenov Y, Rogatsky I: The GRIP1:IRF3 interaction as a target for glucocorticoid receptor-mediated immunosuppression. Embo J 2006;25:108–117.
63 McKay LI, Cidlowski JA: CBP (CREB binding protein) integrates NF-κB (nuclear factor-κB) and glucocorticoid receptor physical interactions and antagonism. Mol Endocrinol 2000; 14:1222–1234.
64 Nissen RM, Yamamoto KR: The glucocorticoid receptor inhibits NFκB by interfering with serine-2 phosphorylation of the RNA polymerase II carboxy-terminal domain. Genes Dev 2000;14:2314–2329.
65 Murphy SH, Suzuki K, Downes M, Welch GL, De Jesus P, Miraglia LJ, Orth AP, Chanda SK, Evans RM, Verma IM: Tumor suppressor protein (p)53, is a regulator of NF-κB repression by the glucocorticoid receptor. Proc Natl AcadSci USA 2011;108:17117–17122.
66 Smoak K, Cidlowski JA: Glucocorticoids regulate tristetraprolin synthesis and posttranscriptionally regulate tumor necrosis factor alpha inflammatory signaling. Mol Cell Biol 2006;26:9126–9135.
67 Carrick DM, Lai WS, Blackshear PJ: The tandem CCCH zinc finger protein tristetraprolin and its relevance to cytokine mRNA turnover and arthritis. Arthritis Res Ther 2004;6:248–264.
68 Dhabhar FS: A hassle a day may keep the doctor away: stress and the augmentation of immune function. Integr Comp Biol 2002;42: 556–564.
69 Chinenov Y, Rogatsky I: Glucocorticoids and the innate immune system: crosstalk with the toll-like receptor signaling network. Mol Cell Endocrinol 2007;275:30–42.
70 Galon J, Franchimont D, Hiroi N, Frey G, Boettner A, Ehrhart-Bornstein M, O'Shea JJ, Chrousos GP, Bornstein SR: Gene profiling reveals unknown enhancing and suppressive actions of glucocorticoids on immune cells. Faseb J 2002;16:61–71.
71 Homma T, Kato A, Hashimoto N, Batchelor J, Yoshikawa M, Imai S, Wakiguchi H, Saito H, Matsumoto K: Corticosteroid and cytokines synergistically enhance toll-like receptor 2 expression in respiratory epithelial cells. Am J Respir Cell Mol Biol 2004;31:463–469.
72 Hermoso MA, Matsuguchi T, Smoak K, Cidlowski JA: Glucocorticoids and tumor necrosis factor alpha cooperatively regulate Toll-like receptor 2 gene expression. Mol Cell Biol 2004;24:4743–4756.
73 Shuto T, Imasato A, Jono H, Sakai A, Xu H, Watanabe T, Rixter DD, Kai H, Andalibi A, Linthicum F, et al: Glucocorticoids synergistically enhance nontypeable *Haemophilus influenzae*-induced Toll-like receptor 2 expression via a negative cross-talk with p38 MAP kinase. J Biol Chem 2002;277:17263–17270.
74 Bornstein SR, Zacharowski P, Schumann RR, Barthel A, Tran N, Papewalis C, Rettori V, McCann SM, Schulze-Osthoff K, Scherbaum WA, et al: Impaired adrenal stress response in Toll-like receptor 2-deficient mice. Proc Natl AcadSci USA 2004;101:16695–16700.
75 Lannan EA, Galliher-Beckley AJ, Scoltock AB, Cidlowski JA: Proinflammatory actions of glucocorticoids: glucocorticoids and TNFα coregulate gene expression in vitro and in vivo. Endocrinology 2012;153:3701–3712.
76 Langlais D, Couture C, Balsalobre A, Drouin J: Regulatory network analyses reveal genome-wide potentiation of LIF signaling by glucocorticoids and define an innate cell defense response. PLoS Genet 2008;4:e1000224.
77 Busillo JM, Azzam KM, Cidlowski JA: Glucocorticoids sensitize the innate immune system through regulation of the NLRP3 inflammasome. J Biol Chem 2011;286:38703–38713.
78 Ding Y, Gao ZG, Jacobson KA, Suffredini AF: Dexamethasone enhances ATP-induced inflammatory responses in endothelial cells. J Pharmacol Exp Ther 2010;335:693–702.
79 Brewer JA, Khor B, Vogt SK, Muglia LM, Fujiwara H, Haegele KE, Sleckman BP, Muglia LJ: T-cell glucocorticoid receptor is required to suppress COX-2-mediated lethal immune activation. Nat Med 2003;9:1318–1322.
80 Kim CJ, Woo YJ, Kim GH, Yoo HW: Familial glucocorticoid deficiency with a point mutation in the ACTH receptor: a case report. J Korean Med Sci 2009;24:979–981.
81 Duma D, Collins JB, Chou JW, Cidlowski JA: Sexually dimorphic actions of glucocorticoids provide a link to inflammatory diseases with gender differences in prevalence. Sci Signal 2010;3:ra74.

NeuroImmunoModulation

Neuroimmunomodulation 2015;22:33–39
DOI: 10.1159/000362733

Published online: September 12, 2014

Circadian Use of Glucocorticoids in Rheumatoid Arthritis

Maurizio Cutolo[a] Alberto Sulli[a] Theodore Pincus[b]

[a]Research Laboratory and Academic Division of Clinical Rheumatology, Department of Internal Medicine, University of Genoa, Genoa, Italy; [b]Rush University, Medical Center, Chicago, Ill., USA

Key Words

Circadian rhythms · Glucocorticoids · Rheumatoid arthritis · Chronotherapy · Cytokines · Melatonin · Sleep · Disease-modifying antirheumatic drugs

Abstract

A clear temporal relationship exists in rheumatoid arthritis (RA) patients between increased nocturnal levels of pro-inflammatory cytokines, such as TNF-α and interleukin (IL)-6, pro-inflammatory hormones (i.e. melatonin, prolactin) and insufficient night production of the anti-inflammatory cortisol (circadian rhythm). Under long-standing chronic stress of disease, insufficient cortisol is available to inhibit an ongoing nocturnal immune/inflammatory reaction. Clinical RA symptoms follow the same circadian rhythm with highest morning severity. Chronotherapy with nighttime glucocorticoid (GC) availability optimizes the treatment of RA patients with low-dose GCs through more efficient targeting of mediators of the immune/inflammatory reaction during the night to be available on arising. Circadian use of low-dose, long-term prednisone, by using night-release formulations (ingested at 10 to 11 p.m.) especially in early RA patients, appears characterized by a significantly superior efficacy on decreasing morning stiffness and IL-6 serum levels, compared to conventional daytime immediate-release prednisone. Shift from medium-dose, immediate-release prednisone (over 7.5–10 mg/day) to night-release formulations GC low-dose, long-term chronotherapy requires a gradual passage, since the hypothalamic-pituitary-adrenal axis of the treated RA patients, potentially altered by a negative feedback induced by the medium/high daily exogenous GC administration, needs time to re-synchronize control of endogenous GC production into a circadian and more physiological nocturnal hormone availability/optimized efficacy.

Chronobiology of Rheumatoid Arthritis

Rheumatoid arthritis (RA) is a multifactorial, immune-mediated and chronic inflammatory syndrome that primarily affects joints, with a circadian clinical symptomatology of inflammation [1]. Some RA patients also experience extra-articular disease, with involvement of lung, thyroid and/or exocrine glands, and/or other organs. The early use of disease-modifying antirheumatic drugs (DMARDs), particularly methotrexate, and the availability of new biologic therapies targeted to inflammatory cytokines or extra- and intra-cellular signaling mediators have improved RA management significantly over the last 3 decades [2].

Low-dose glucocorticoids (GCs) have been found to be effective not only in relieving the signs and symptoms of RA, but also in slowing radiographic progression, gen-

KARGER

E-Mail karger@karger.com
www.karger.com/nim

1021–7401/14/0222–0033$39.50/0

Maurizio Cutolo, MD
Research Laboratories and Academic Division of Clinical Rheumatology
Department of Internal Medicine, University of Genoa, Viale Benedetto XV, 6
IT–16132 Genoa (Italy)
E-Mail mcutolo@unige.it

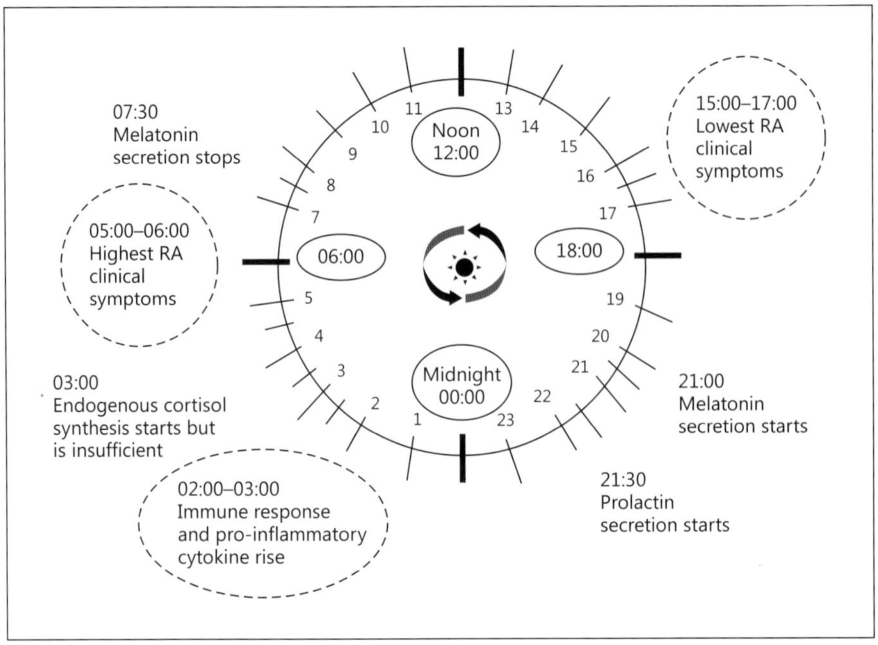

Fig. 1. In RA patients, a clear temporal relationship exists early in the night between increased nocturnal levels of pro-inflammatory cytokines (such as TNF-α and IL-6) and pro-inflammatory hormones (such as melatonin and prolactin), and the insufficient night production of the endogenous anti-inflammatory cortisol which, under chronic stress of disease, becomes insufficient to inhibit the ongoing nocturnal immune/inflammatory reaction. The clinical consequence is the highest clinical morning symptomatology in RA patients.

erally in combination with synthetic DMARDs [3–6]. GCs may elicit different types of biological responses, including adverse effects, depending on cell targets, dosages, time of administration and other variables [7, 8]. The anti-inflammatory and immunosuppressive effects of GCs are well characterized. Nonetheless, their mode of action is highly complex and involves extensive neuroendocrine networks [9].

Symptoms of RA, such as fatigue, joint pain, swelling and morning stiffness, display pronounced circadian rhythms, with the highest severity in the early morning [10, 11] (fig. 1). Therefore, in RA patients, a clear temporal relationship exists between increased nocturnal levels of pro-inflammatory cytokines [such as TNF-α and interleukin (IL)-6] and pro-inflammatory hormones (such as melatonin and prolactin), and insufficient night production of endogenous anti-inflammatory cortisol. Under chronic stress of disease, cortisol is not sufficient to inhibit ongoing nocturnal immune/inflammatory reactions [12, 13] (fig. 1).

As a result, the current most advanced approach to optimize the risk-benefit ratio for long-term GC treatment in RA involves low-dose chronotherapy with night-release prednisone (available in the late night). A similar chronotherapeutic approach may also be effective with the use of DMARDs like methotrexate and non-steroidal anti-inflammatory drugs (NSAIDs).

Sleep, Cortisol and Chronobiology

The crucial role of sleep, which is an important condition for the homoeostatic regulation of chronobiological processes of the immune network, is a matter of considerable research [14, 15]. Uncoupling or dysregulation of the cortisol circadian rhythm under the influence of the central nervous CLOCK (Circadian Locomotor Output Cycles Kaput) system (darkness, light alternation), and local tissue sensitivity to GCs by the peripheral CLOCK, may induce a tissue functional hypercortisolism, which could be followed by the development of pathologic conditions, including dysregulation of the immune system and metabolic disturbaces [16].

Individuals exposed to conditions that induce a dysregulation of cortisol circadian rhythm include rotating shift workers, whose circadian system is repetitively reset by nighttime activity and daytime sleep, or individuals exposed to frequent jet lag from travel over many time zones [17, 18] (fig. 2). As a consequence, these subjects are at an increased risk of developing various pathologic conditions, such as components of the metabolic syndrome or cardiometabolic disease and stroke, which might result from increased target tissue exposure to GCs (secondary hypercortisolism) [19].

Conversely, prolonged sleep loss, as induced for example by sleep restriction, produces a stress-like response (a chronic-like stress condition with reduced cortisol availability) which is characterized immunologically by inflammation, with increases in pro-inflammatory cytokine serum levels such as IL-6 and related C-reactive protein elevation [20]. Recently, Ramadan followers were found to have abolished cortisol circadian rhythm and their circulating insulin levels and HOMA (homeostasis model assessment) index were found to be increased during this period, which is associated with disturbed feeding and sleep patterns [21].

Clearly, a major candidate for the effects of sleep deprivation in any individual is cortisol, the most potent hormone involved in the stress-response system. Cortisol increases sequentially the production, bone marrow release, intravascular half-life and demargination of neutrophils, which are also involved in immune/inflammatory responses [22]. Therefore, a long-term altered cortisol night rhythm, together with mediators that are known to be regulated by sleep and the circadian system, including melatonin, prolactin, growth hormone, leptin, vitamin D and vasopressin, may contribute to a pro-inflammatory state induced during nocturnal sleep [14] (fig. 2).

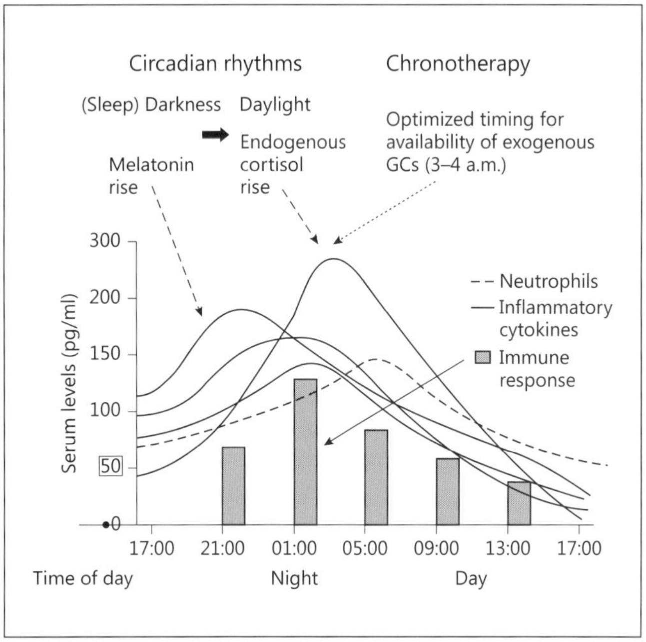

Fig. 2. Exogenous GCs are recommended at low doses and as long-term treatment in chronic inflammatory diseases (such as RA) and may act as 'replacement' therapy (rather than 'pharmacologic' therapy) in the presence of decreased endogenous cortisol availability due to the chronicity of the disease. The current most advanced approach to improve the risk-benefit ratio of GCs is low-dose exogenous prednisone chronotherapy with modified-release prednisone, a timed drug release (releasing prednisone at 3 a.m.) to modulate the chronobiological rhythms of inflammation.

Mediators of Circadian Clinical Symptoms in Arthritis

Symptoms of RA, such as morning stiffness, show a clear temporal relationship with nocturnally elevated levels of pro-inflammatory cytokines, as a consequence of a cascade of increased nocturnal inflammation [10]. Several of these cytokines, such as TNF-α and IL-6, are highly increased in patients with active RA in the early hours of the day, but are found at very low levels after noon [23]. Their release pattern and serum concentrations, possibly triggered by pro-inflammatory hormones such as melatonin (and prolactin), follow a 24-hour daily cycle [24].

As noted, these pro-inflammatory hormones begin to rise before the onset of RA symptoms, and before activation of endogenous cortisol synthesis that counteracts the cascade of the immune/inflammatory processes [10]. In addition, rhythmic fluctuations of the nocturnal secretion and the peripheral metabolism of endogenous cortisol, as well as changes in the activation of biologically inactive to active cortisone in the synovial cells (intracrinology), appear important in the pathophysiology of RA [11].

Therefore, the RA inflammatory process induces changes in synovial fluid composition, edema of synovial tissue, as well as a redistribution of interstitial fluid, while sleeping contributes to clinical stiffness of the joints that is most pronounced in the early morning [25]. All these processes are closely linked to regulatory interactions between the endocrine, nervous and immune systems, with distinct 24-hour daily rhythms [25].

While the role of IL-6 and TNF-α in the regulation of inflammatory and immune responses, particularly in RA, is well established, the increased production of other pro-inflammatory cytokines, such as IL-8, IL-12 and IL-17, by primary and secondary immune cells may also be implicated in the circadian process [26]. Furthermore, in polymyalgia rheumatica (PMR), symptoms of pain and stiffness are typically most prominent during the early morning, similar to RA [27]. There are indications for circadian variation of TNF-α and IL-6 secretion with peak values in the early morning hours. Therefore, given the known high GC sensitivity of PMR, time-adapted GC therapy can be hypothesized to be likely more effective than the currently used standard regimen in improving clinical symptoms [27–30].

Of note, in another inflammatory arthritic condition, namely ankylosing spondylitis, pain and stiffness also seem to be most prominent during the early morning hours [27]. Finally, it is now also evident that symptoms of diseases such as RA, which is T helper 1 dependent, but also asthma, which is T helper 2 dependent, are influenced by diurnal rhythms and natural regulatory T cells [31]. In particular, secretion of IL-2, IFN-γ and IL-10 by naïve CD4+ T cells follows a diurnal rhythm [31].

The Circadian Use Optimizes GC Treatment of RA and Adrenal Insufficiency

Exogenous GCs are recommended at low doses and as long-term treatment in chronic inflammatory diseases (i.e. RA or systemic lupus erythematosus), and may act as 'replacement' therapy (rather than 'pharmacologic' therapy) in the presence of decreased endogenous cortisol availability due to the chronicity of the disease [32, 33] (fig. 2). When used in high doses, even greater than 10 mg/day over long periods, exogenous GCs may induce adverse effects, which may be reduced by considering the endogenous rhythm of synthesis that begins to rise in the early hours of the morning (between 2 and 4 a.m.), peaks around 6 to 8 a.m. and has a nadir around 10 p.m. to 2 a.m. [34].

GCs exert important genomic effects on cellular immunity that, in concert with cellular circadian rhythms, reduce or prevent night upregulation of immune cell activity (and the related flare of cytokine synthesis) with administration of exogenous GCs between 6 and 8 a.m., which may not be optimal given the existence of cellular circadian rhythms [35]. Since pain, stiffness and functional disability show maximum symptoms in the early morning hours in RA patients, preceded by elevated serum levels of IL-6 (which is also an adrenal gland activator), preventing the nocturnal rise of pro-inflammatory cytokines by GC therapy is more effective than treating the morning symptoms (i.e. morning stiffness and pain) [36]. The current most advanced approach to improve the risk-benefit ratio of GCs is the low-dose prednisone chronotherapy with modified-release prednisone, a timing drug release (releasing prednisone at 3 a.m.) to modulate the chronobiological rhythms of inflammation [37, 38] (fig. 2).

Two large-scale trials documented that modified-release prednisone has a greater efficacy for long-term, low-dose GC treatment in RA patients, showing a significant reduction in morning joint stiffness, in addition to all known therapeutic effects with conventional prednisone and a similar safety profile but without additional suppression of the hypothalamic-pituitary-adrenal (HPA) axis, as observed for immediate-release prednisone at 7.5 mg [39–42]. Therefore, the specific timing of prednisone, linked to the interaction between IL-6 and the HPA axis, may correct a postulated deficiency in HPA control in RA [29].

The proliferation of the cells involved in the RA immune/inflammatory response represents an important target for disease-modifying treatment (with DMARDs), and the administration of recommended anti-proliferative/anti-inflammatory drugs (i.e. methotrexate, leflunomide, cyclophosphamide, etc.) might follow the same concepts of GC chronotherapy [2]. This hypothesis was recently tested in an in vivo investigation using an animal model of arthritis, which showed that the optimal dosing time, associated with the 24-hour cycling of TNF-α, could lead to optimization of methotrexate anti-inflammatory action (and decrease of TNF-α) [43]. A further clinical study confirmed that bedtime methotrexate chronotherapy (3 times a week once a day) can improve RA symptoms compared to the current usual weekly dosing methods [44].

A recent clinical study strengthened the belief that reproducing circadian cortisol levels in adrenal insufficiency (a condition resulting from severe RA or PMR adrenal failure) may improve quality of life by using the circadian hydrocortisone replacement [45]. Treating patients with a modified-release preparation of hydrocortisone (i.e. Chronocort) has been found to simulate the overnight rise in cortisol release, obtaining a single peak level at 6 a.m. [45]. More recently, patients with adrenal insufficiency were treated with modified-release prednisone and showed decreased complaints and fatigue compared to standard prednisolone, again indicating the importance of GC increase/availability in the very early morning hours, before waking [46].

Practical Clinical Issues Arising from the Use of Modified-Release Prednisone in RA

The earliest use of a GC agent with modified release in inflammatory conditions occurred almost 15 years ago, with the potent GC budesonide (formulated to dissolve in a pH-dependent manner). This approach was found to provide an effective form of therapy for the treatment of Crohn's disease located in the distal ileum, ileocecal region and ascending colon [47]. Modified release of Budesonide was found to have effectiveness equal to or less than that of prednisolone or prednisone therapy in the treatment of active Crohn's disease, but was associated with fewer GC adverse reactions [47].

The modified release of prednisone 4–5 h after ingestion has been available for 5 years. Recently, single-center crossover studies were conducted, each in ≤24 healthy subjects, to compare the pharmacokinetics of a single 5-mg oral dose of modified-release prednisone and conventional prednisone, as well as the effect of food on bioavailability [48]. There was no substantial difference in pharmacokinetic parameters of the formulations apart from the programmed delay in release of GC from the modified-release tablets.

Administration after a full or light meal did not affect pharmacokinetic characteristics, but bioavailability was reduced under fasting conditions. Pharmacokinetic evaluation in 9 patients with RA confirmed that modified-release prednisone tablets taken at bedtime with or after an evening meal result in programmed release of GC 4–6 h after intake [49].

Recently, as mentioned, the effects of long-term, low-dose chronotherapy with modified-release prednisone on the HPA axis have been investigated in RA patients [39]. The mean increase of cortisol plasma concentrations after injection of corticorelin was 5.5 (SD 4.37) μg/dl on regular prednisone at baseline and 5.3 (4.07) μg/dl on modified-release prednisone at 12 months.

The number of normal, suppressed and no response reactions did not differ among treatments. Switching from regular to modified-release prednisone did not influence responses, nor did long-term treatment of up to 12 months with modified-release GC [39]. Finally, no worsening of adrenal impairment was observed on treatment with nighttime-release prednisone in patients with low responsiveness to corticotropin-releasing hormone testing before the treatment with such approach.

A very recent observational study assessed the functional ability in RA patients treated with modified release prednisone under conditions of normal clinical practice [50]. Interestingly, the dose of night-available prednisone was significantly reduced after 9 months of treatment (from 5.0 to 4.4 mg/day, $p < 0.001$) and fewer RA patients required biological treatments, analgesia and gastroprotectants. In long-term, low-dose GC therapy (lasting years), a possible progressive dose decrease might be biologically meaningful.

In order to verify whether modified-release prednisone taken at bedtime was superior with respect to the improvement of morning symptoms compared to immediate-release prednisone taken in the morning, 950 RA outpatients treated with different DMARDs (83.7% methotrexate, 10.5% leflunomide; 15.8% biologics) and medium- to low-dose GCs were switched from immediate-release prednisone or 6-methyl-prednisolone to low-dose, modified-release prednisone and followed for 4 months [50]. In particular, 513 RA patients were switched to modified-release prednisone from immediate-release prednisone (9.4 ± 5.4 mg) and 437 from 6-methyl-prednisolone (6.7 ± 3.7 mg).

Among 920 patients (96.8%) completing 4 months of modified-release prednisone treatment, morning stiffness duration, pain intensity (numerical rating scale 0–10), patient and physician global assessment and disease activity score (DAS28) improved significantly ($p < 0.001$) [50]. Mean daily modified-release prednisone dosage again decreased from 8.2 to 6.7 mg between baseline and endpoint. In summary, even if GC-naïve RA patients have been found to be better responders to the modified-release prednisone, switching daytime GC-treated RA patients to low-dose modified-release prednisone seems to improve outcomes significantly over 4 months [50].

Cost-Effectiveness Issues of Modified-Release Prednisone in RA Treatment

After having assessed the safety and effectiveness of prednisone chronotherapy with new modified-release formulations, it is important to evaluate cost-effectiveness. This is particularly relevant in RA due to the chronic nature of the disease, rising management costs, which are especially increased with the high cost of biologic agents, and budget-constrained healthcare systems.

A recent UK study used a health state transition model to categorize RA patients into four health states, based on the duration of morning stiffness [51]. The model applied a 1-year time horizon and adopted a UK National Health Service perspective. Health benefits were evaluated as quality-adjusted life years (QALY) and the final output was the incremental cost-effectiveness ratio. Efficacy data were derived from the original study on modified-release prednisone study, drug costs from the British National Formulary, and utility data from a direct elicitation time-trade-off study in the general population [17, 51].

As expected, mean treatment costs per patient were found to be higher for modified-release (GBP 649.70) than for immediate-release prednisone (GBP 46.54) for the duration of the model. However, the model generated an incremental QALY of 0.044 in favor of modified-release prednisone, which resulted in an incremental cost-effectiveness ratio of GBP 13,577. These results must be confirmed by further studies.

Probabilistic sensitivity analysis reported that modified-release prednisone had an 84% probability of being cost-effective at a willingness-to-pay threshold of GBP 30,000 per QALY and is a cost-effective treatment option [51].

In another recent study, the effects of a 12-week treatment with modified-release prednisone versus placebo on the costs of drug treatment of RA were modeled [52]. The results showed 11–13% more patients on modified-release prednisone than on placebo dropped below reimbursement thresholds for the Netherlands, Belgium and the UK. Assuming 1 year of biologics cost EUR 15,000 and modified-release prednisone costs EUR 1/day, almost EUR 396 should be saved in each RA patient by delaying biologic treatment by 12 weeks (where possible). The conclusion again is that despite a considerably higher cost than conventional prednisone, modified-release prednisone is a cost-effective option for RA patients not on GCs who are eligible for therapy with biologic agents.

Conclusions

Chronotherapy with night-time GC availability optimizes the use of low-dose GCs in RA patients, and also possibly of DMARDs and NSAIDs (at least at bedtime), through a more efficient targeting of the mediators of the immune/inflammatory reaction during their night rising time [43, 53–55]. These results were anticipated almost 30 years ago by the direct night administration of prednisone to RA patients; however, the system was not introduced to clinical practice because it was not practical to administer GCs to patients at 3–4 a.m. [56–58].

Circadian use of low-dose, long-term prednisone by using night-release formulations (ingested at 10–11 p.m.) especially in GC-naïve RA patients is characterized by a significantly superior effectiveness, at least on morning symptoms and IL-6 serum level reduction, when compared to conventional daytime immediate-release prednisone [40, 59]. Of note, the shift from medium-dose, immediate-release prednisone (over 7.5–10 mg/day) to night-release formulations GC low-dose, long-term chronotherapy requires a gradual passage, since the HPA axis of the treated RA patients (non-GC naïve), potentially altered by a negative feedback induced by the medium/high daily exogenous GC administration, needs time to re-synchronize control of endogenous GC production into a circadian and more physiological nocturnal hormone availability/optimized efficacy [39, 42]. However, the safety of low-dose prednisone regarding HPA function was already assessed 20 years ago [60] and, in particular, spontaneous recovery of the HPA axis was found to be usual for patients who are taking prednisone at daily doses of 5 mg or less [60].

References

1 McInnes IB, O'Dell JR: State-of-the-art: rheumatoid arthritis. Ann Rheum Dis 2010;69:1898–1906.
2 Smolen JS, Landewé R, Breedveld FC, et al: EULAR recommendations for the management of rheumatoid arthritis with synthetic and biological disease-modifying antirheumatic drugs: 2013 update. Ann Rheum Dis 2014;73:492–509.
3 Bakker MF, Jacobs JW, Welsing PM, et al: Low-dose prednisone inclusion in a methotrexate-based, tight control strategy for early rheumatoid arthritis: a randomized trial. Ann Intern Med 2012;156:329–339.
4 Gorter SL, Bijlsma JW, Cutolo M, et al: Current evidence for the management of rheumatoid arthritis with glucocorticoids: a systematic literature review informing the EULAR recommendations for the management of rheumatoid arthritis. Ann Rheum Dis 2010;69:1010–1014.
5 Pincus T, Sokka T, Castrejón I, et al: Decline of mean initial prednisone dosage from 10.3 to 3.6 mg/day to treat rheumatoid arthritis between 1980 and 2004 in one clinical setting, with long-term effectiveness of dosages less than 5 mg/day. Arthritis Care Res (Hoboken) 2013;65:729–736.
6 Wassenberg S, Rau R, Steinfeld P, et al: Very low-dose prednisolone in early rheumatoid arthritis retards radiographic progression over two years: a multicenter, double-blind, placebo-controlled trial. Arthritis Rheum 2005;52:3371–3380.
7 van der Goes MC, Jacobs JW, Boers M, et al: Patient and rheumatologist perspectives on glucocorticoids: an exercise to improve the implementation of the European League Against Rheumatism (EULAR) recommendations on the management of systemic glucocorticoid therapy in rheumatic diseases. Ann Rheum Dis 2010;69:1015–1021.
8 Strehl C, Spies CM, Buttgereit F: Pharmacodynamics of glucocorticoids. Clin Exp Rheumatol 2011;29(5 suppl 68):S13–S18.
9 Cutolo M, Buttgereit F, Straub RH: Regulation of glucocorticoids by the central nervous system. Clin Exp Rheumatol 2011;29(5 suppl 68):S19–S22.
10 Sierakowski S, Cutolo M: Morning symptoms in rheumatoid arthritis: a defining characteristic and marker of active disease. Scand J Rheumatol Suppl 2011;125:1–5.
11 Cutolo M: Rheumatoid arthritis: circadian and circannual rhythms in RA. Nat Rev Rheumatol 2011;7:500–502.
12 Straub RH, Cutolo M: Effects of the neuroendocrine system on development and function of the immune system; in Hochberg MC, Silman AJ, Smolen JS, Weinblatt ME, Weisman MH (eds): Rheumatology, ed 5. Amsterdam, Elsevier, 2014, chap 25.
13 Crofford LJ, Kalogeras KT, Mastorakos G, et al: Circadian relationships between interleukin (IL)-6 and hypothalamic-pituitary-adrenal axis hormones: failure of IL-6 to cause sustained hypercortisolism in patients with early untreated rheumatoid arthritis. J Clin Endocrinol Metab 1997;82:1279–1283.

14 Lange T, Dimitrov S, Born J: Effects of sleep and circadian rhythm on the human immune system. Ann NY Acad Sci 2010;1193:48–59.
15 Straub RH, Cutolo M, Buttgereit F, et al: Energy regulation and neuroendocrine-immune control in chronic inflammatory diseases. J Intern Med 2010;267:543–560.
16 Chrousos GP: The hypothalamic-pituitary-adrenal axis and immune-mediated inflammation. N Engl J Med 1995;332:1351–1362.
17 Haus EL, Smolensky MH: Shift work and cancer risk: potential mechanistic roles of circadian disruption, light at night, and sleep deprivation. Sleep Med Rev 2013;17:273–284.
18 Doane LD, Kremen WS, Eaves LJ, et al: Associations between jet lag and cortisol diurnal rhythms after domestic travel. Health Psychol 2010;29:117–123.
19 Kino T, Chrousos GP: Acetylation-mediated epigenetic regulation of glucocorticoid receptor activity: circadian rhythm-associated alterations of glucocorticoid actions in target tissues. Mol Cell Endocrinol 2011;336:23–30.
20 Pejovic S, Basta M, Vgontzas AN, et al: Effects of recovery sleep after one work week of mild sleep restriction on interleukin-6 and cortisol secretion and daytime sleepiness and performance. Am J Physiol Endocrinol Metab 2013;305:E890–E896.
21 Bahijri S, Borai A, Ajabnoor G, et al: Relative metabolic stability, but disrupted circadian cortisol secretion during the fasting month of Ramadan. PLoS One 2013;8:e60917.
22 Mullington JM, Haack M, Toth M, et al: Cardiovascular, inflammatory, and metabolic consequences of sleep deprivation. Prog Cardiovasc Dis 2009;51:294–302.
23 Straub RH, Bijlsma JW, Masi A, et al: Role of neuroendocrine and neuroimmune mechanisms in chronic inflammatory rheumatic diseases: the 10-year update. Semin Arthritis Rheum 2013;43:392–404.
24 Cutolo M: Chronobiology and the treatment of rheumatoid arthritis. Curr Opin Rheumatol 2012;24:312–318.
25 Cutolo M, Straub RH, Bijlsma JW: Neuroendocrine-immune interactions in synovitis. Nat Clin Pract Rheumatol 2007;3:627–634.
26 Cutolo M, Straub RH: Circadian rhythms in arthritis: hormonal effects on the immune/inflammatory reaction. Autoimmun Rev 2008;7:223–228.
27 Spies CM, Cutolo M, Straub RH, et al: More night than day – circadian rhythms in polymyalgia rheumatica and ankylosing spondylitis. J Rheumatol 2010;37:894–899.
28 Caporali R, Cimmino MA, Montecucco C, et al: Glucocorticoid treatment of polymyalgia rheumatica. Clin Exp Rheumatol 2011;29(5 suppl 68):S143–S147.
29 Cutolo M, Foppiani L, Minuto F: Hypothalamic-pituitary-adrenal axis impairment in the pathogenesis of rheumatoid arthritis and polymyalgia rheumatica. J Endocrinol Invest 2002;25(10 suppl):19–23.
30 Straub RH, Gluck T, Cutolo M, et al: The adrenal steroid status in relation to inflammatory cytokines (interleukin-6 and tumour necrosis factor) in polymyalgia rheumatica. Rheumatology 2000;39:624–631.
31 Bollinger T, Bollinger A, Naujoks J, et al: The influence of regulatory T cells and diurnal hormone rhythms on T helper cell activity. Immunology 2010;131:488–500.
32 Buttgereit F, Burmester GR, Straub RH, et al: Exogenous and endogenous glucocorticoids in rheumatic diseases. Arthritis Rheum 2011;63:1–9.
33 Gorter SL, Bijlsma JW, Cutolo M, et al: Current evidence for the management of rheumatoid arthritis with glucocorticoids: a systematic literature review informing the EULAR recommendations for the management of rheumatoid arthritis. Ann Rheum Dis 2010;69:1010–1014.
34 van der Goes MC, Jacobs JW, Boers M, et al: Monitoring adverse events of low-dose glucocorticoid therapy: EULAR recommendations for clinical trials and daily practice. Ann Rheum Dis 2010;69:1913–1919.
35 Cutolo M, Seriolo B, Craviotto C, et al: Circadian rhythms in RA. Ann Rheum Dis 2003;62:593–596.
36 Cutolo M, Otsa K, Aakre O, et al: Nocturnal hormones and clinical rhythms in rheumatoid arthritis. Ann NY Acad Sci 2005;1051:372–381.
37 Jacobs JW, Bijlsma JW: Modified release prednisone in patients with rheumatoid arthritis. Ann Rheum Dis 2010;69:1257–1259.
38 Spies CM, Cutolo M, Straub RH, et al: Prednisone chronotherapy. Clin Exp Rheumatol 2011;29(5 suppl 68):S42–S45.
39 Alten R, Döring G, Cutolo M, et al: Hypothalamus-pituitary-adrenal axis function in patients with rheumatoid arthritis treated with nighttime-release prednisone. J Rheumatol 2010;37:2025–2031.
40 Buttgereit F, Doering G, Shaeffler A, et al: Efficacy of modified-release versus standard prednisone to reduce duration of morning stiffness of the joints in rheumatoid arthritis (CAPRA-1): a double-blind, randomised controlled trial. Lancet 2008;371:205–214.
41 Buttgereit F, Doering G, Schaeffler A, et al: Targeting pathophysiological rhythms: prednisone chronotherapy shows sustained efficacy in rheumatoid arthritis. Ann Rheum Dis 2010;69:1275–1280.
42 Kirwan JR, Hickey SH, Hällgren R, et al: The effect of therapeutic glucocorticoids on the adrenal response in a randomized controlled trial in patients with rheumatoid arthritis. Arthritis Rheum 2006;54:1415–1421.
43 To H, Irie S, Tomonari M, et al: Therapeutic index of methotrexate depends on circadian cycling of tumour necrosis factor-α in collagen-induced arthritic rats and mice. J Pharm Pharmacol 2009;61:1333–1338.
44 To H, Yoshimatsu H, Tomonari M, Ida H, et al: Methotrexate chronotherapy is effective against rheumatoid arthritis. Chronobiol Int 2011;28:267–274.
45 Debbono M, Ross RJ: Optimal glucocorticoid therapy. Endocr Dev 2011;20:173–180.
46 Langenheim J, Ventz M, Hinz A, et al: Modified-release prednisone decreases complaints and fatigue compared to standard prednisolone in patients with adrenal insufficiency. Horm Metab Res 2013;45:96–101.
47 Baker DE: Budesonide modified-release capsules. Rev Gastroenterol Disord 2001;1:147–155.
48 Derendorf H, Ruebsamen K, Clarke L, et al: Pharmacokinetics of modified-release prednisone tablets in healthy subjects and patients with rheumatoid arthritis. J Clin Pharmacol 2013;53:326–333.
49 Pfeiffer BM, Krenzer S, Dockhorn R, et al: Impact of modified-release prednisone on functional ability in patients with rheumatoid arthritis. Rheumatol Int 2013;33:1447–1454.
50 Cutolo M, Iaccarino L, Doria A, et al: Efficacy of the switch to modified-release prednisone in rheumatoid arthritis patients treated with standard glucocorticoids. Clin Exp Rheumatol 2013;31:498–505.
51 Dunlop W, Iqbal I, et al: Cost-effectiveness of modified-release prednisone in the treatment of moderate to severe rheumatoid arthritis with morning stiffness based on directly elicited public preference values. Clinicoecon Outcomes Res 2013;5:555–564.
52 Boers M, Buttgereit F: A simple model that suggests possible cost savings when modified-release prednisone 5 mg/day is added to current treatment in patients with active rheumatoid arthritis. Rheumatology (Oxford) 2013;52:1435–1437.
53 Pincus T, Castrejon I, Yazici Y: Low-dose prednisone inclusion in a methotrexate-based, tight control strategy for early rheumatoid arthritis. Ann Intern Med 2012;157:299.
54 Levi F, Le Louarn C, Reinberg A: Timing optimizes sustained-release indomethacin treatment of osteoarthritis. Clin Pharmacol Ther 1985;37:77–84.
55 Pincus T, Bijlsma JW, Braun J, et al: Low-dose glucocorticoids in rheumatic diseases: introduction. Clin Exp Rheumatol 2011;29(5 suppl 68):S2–S4.
56 De Silva M, Binder A, Hazleman BL: The timing of prednisolone dosage and its effect on morning stiffness in rheumatoid arthritis. Ann Rheum Dis 1984;43:790–793.
57 Arvidson NG, Gudbjörnsson B, Elfman L, et al: Circadian rhythm of serum interleukin-6 in rheumatoid arthritis. Ann Rheum Dis 1994;53:521–524.
58 Arvidson NG, Gudbjornsson B, Larsson A, et al: The timing of glucocorticoid administration in rheumatoid arthritis. Ann Rheum Dis 1997;56:27–31.
59 Da Silva JA: Safety of glucocorticoids – clinical trials. Clin Exp Rheumatol 2011;29(5 suppl 68):S99–S103.
60 LaRochelle GE Jr, LaRochelle AG, Ratner RE, Borenstein DG: Recovery of the hypothalamic-pituitary-adrenal (HPA) axis in patients with rheumatic diseases receiving low-dose prednisone. Am J Med 1993;95:258–264.

NeuroImmunoModulation

Neuroimmunomodulation 2015;22:40–45
DOI: 10.1159/000362725

Published online: September 12, 2014

11β-Hydroxysteroid Dehydrogenase Enzymes Modulate Effects of Glucocorticoids in Rheumatoid Arthritis Synovial Cells

Martin Schmidt[a] Rainer H. Straub[b]

[a]Institute of Biochemistry II, Jena University Hospital, Friedrich Schiller University Jena, Jena, and [b]Laboratory of Experimental Rheumatology and Neuroendocrine Immunology, Department of Internal Medicine I, University Hospital Regensburg, Regensburg, Germany

Key Words

Rheumatoid arthritis · Glucocorticoid receptor · 11β-Hydroxysteroid dehydrogenases

Abstract

The tissue availability of active glucocorticoids (cortisol in humans) depends on their rate of synthesis from cholesterol, downstream metabolism, excretion and interconversion. The latter is mediated by the 11β-hydroxysteroid dehydrogenases (11βHSDs). In this review, we summarize the features of the two isoenzymes, 11βHSD1 and 11βHSD2, and current available experimental data related to 11βHSDs, which are relevant in the context of synovial cells in rheumatoid arthritis (RA). We conclude that due to complex feedback mechanisms inherent to the hypothalamic-pituitary-adrenal axis, currently available transgenic animal models cannot display the full potential otherwise inherent to the techniques. Studies with tissue explants, mixed synovial cell preparations, cell lines derived from synovial cells, and related primary cells or established cell lines indicate that there are relatively clear differences between the two isoenzymes. 11βHSD1 is expressed primarily in fibroblasts and osteoblasts, and may be responsible for fibroblast survival and aid in the resolution of inflammation, but it is also involved in bone damage. 11βHSD2 is expressed primarily in macrophages and lymphocytes, and may be responsible for their survival, suggesting that it is critical in chronic inflammation. The situation in synovial tissue would allow 11βHSD2-expressing cells to tap the energy resources of 11βHSD1-expressing cells. The overall properties of this local glucocorticoid interconversion system might limit therapeutic use of glucocorticoids in RA.

Introduction

The sheer number of papers (almost 8,000), which can be found in a PubMed search using the search string '(glucocorticoid OR cortisone OR cortisol OR prednisone OR prednisolone OR dexamethasone) AND rheumatoid arthritis', indicate that the introduction of glucocorticoids into the treatment of rheumatoid arthritis (RA) by Hench et al. [1] must be considered a success. In the late 1960s, a role for peripheral cortisone-cortisol interconversion in RA was described [2] and involvement of synovial tissue in this interconversion was shown [3]. However, more detailed elucidation of the underlying mechanisms was possible only after the necessary techniques became available [4].

KARGER

E-Mail karger@karger.com
www.karger.com/nim

1021–7401/14/0222–0040$39.50/0

Prof. Dr. Rainer H. Straub
Laboratory of Experimental Rheumatology and Neuroendocrine Immunology
Department of Internal Medicine I, University Hospital, BIOPARK 1
Josef-Engert-Strasse 9, DE–93053 Regensburg (Germany)
E-Mail rainer.straub@ukr.de

11β-Hydroxysteroid Dehydrogenases

The principle biochemical pathways involved in glucocorticoid synthesis from cholesterol, their interconversion, their downstream metabolism and their excretion are known (fig. 1) and have been described in excellent reviews [5, 6]. It is now evident that the effects of the endogenous glucocorticoids, as well as therapeutic drugs, depend critically on the intra-tissue activities of the enzymes involved in their interconversion, the 11β-hydroxysteroid dehydrogenases (11βHSDs) [7].

In humans, there exist two 11βHSD isoenzymes (EC 1.1.1.146), which are encoded by separate genes and catalyze remarkably different reactions. The type 1 enzyme (11βHSD1) is encoded by the gene HSD11B1 and predominantly mediates the conversion of 11-oxosteroids to their corresponding 11β-hydroxysteroids using NADPH as a cofactor, but might work in a reverse mode under certain circumstances [8, 9]. By contrast, the type 2 enzyme (11βHSD2) is encoded by the gene HSD11B2 and exclusively mediates the conversion of 11β-hydroxysteroids to their corresponding 11-oxosteroids using NAD^+ as a cofactor [10, 11].

Although their most prominent physiological roles are the reactivation of cortisone into the glucocorticoid receptor (GR) agonist cortisol (11βHSD1) and the inactivation of cortisol into the biologically inactive cortisone (11βHSD2), both enzymes can metabolize various additional substrates with similar structures. Generally, these additional substrates are not prominent, but in principle all steroidal substances containing 11-keto/11-hydroxy functional groups can compete with the endogenous corticosteroids for the catalytically active sites of the 11βHSDs [12]. Among these are prednisone or prednisolone, as well as some 7-keto/7-hydroxy cholesterol metabolites, which are sterically similar to normal 11βHSD substrates [9, 13]. Moreover, these metabolites can compete with glucocorticoids for the 11βHSDs active sites [14], which may result in alterations of net conversion rates of cortisol and cortisone, respectively, strongly depending on the concentrations of alternative substrates within a given tissue.

In line with their opposing catalytic activities, expression of both 11βHSD isoenzymes seems to follow simple rules. 11βHSD1 expression levels are highest in tissues where the GR signaling is important, e.g. in the liver [7, 8]. In contrast, 11βHSD2 expression is strong in tissues in which either GR activation should be avoided or glucocorticoids would interfere with specific mineralocorticoid signaling, e.g. in the kidney [7, 10, 11, 15]. This dual function of 11βHSD2 was shown in detail in a study in human fetal tissues by Condon et al. [16]. In addition, overexpression of 11βHSD2 in pituitary tumors was shown to be at least in part responsible for cell proliferation [17].

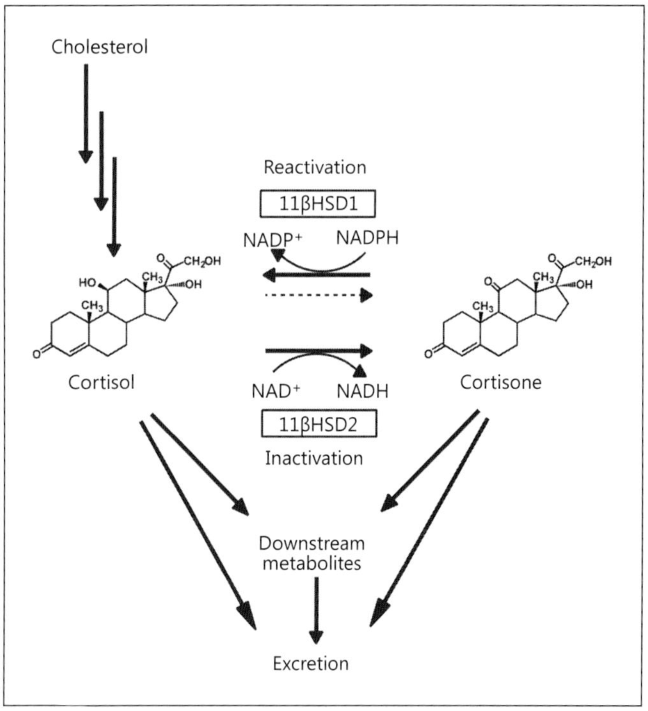

Fig. 1. Pathways involved in glucocorticoid metabolism. Glucocorticoid synthesis from cholesterol, downstream metabolism and excretion are summarized by arrows. The reactions catalyzed by the two 11βHSD isoforms are shown. The dashed arrow indicates the backward reaction seen only for purified 11βHSD1 in vitro.

Lessons Learned and Not (Yet) Learned from Animal Models

Transgenic animal models can yield valuable information to elucidate the roles of individual genes or proteins. Accordingly, available mice with targeted inactivation (knock-out) of 11βHSDs were soon analyzed for phenotypic alterations related to inflammatory diseases [reviewed in 18]: mice without 11βHSD1 exhibit a complex but subtle inflammatory phenotype. More recently, it was shown that lack of 11βHSD1 exaggerates inflammation in various mouse models of experimental arthritis [19]. In a rat arthritis model, inhibition of local glucocorticoid reactivation by 11βHSD1, as well as inhibition of GR signaling by RU486, increased inflammatory paw volume (as

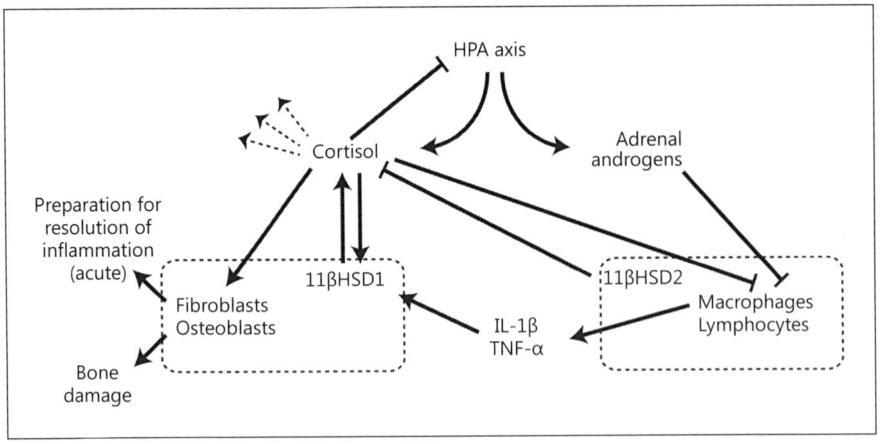

Fig. 2. 11βHSDs modulate the amount of cortisol and its effects. The amount of cortisol (the active glucocorticoid) depends on the functional HPA axis and the activities of the two 11βHSD isoenzymes: 11βHSD1 increases cortisol and 11βHSD2 reduces cortisol; too much cortisol inhibits the HPA axis and reduces the anti-inflammatory androgens. This becomes critical in cells not responding to cortisol because of 11βHSD2 expression. Arrows indicate synthesis, induction or activation; blunted lines indicate degradation or inhibition.

readout for inflammation) [20]. But generally the phenotypes seen in these experiments are associated with adrenal hyperplasia and elevated systemic corticosterone levels (the active glucocorticoid in rodents), which seem to compensate for the absence of local reactivation of glucocorticoids by 11βHSD1.

This is mirrored in humans, in whom reduced 11βHSD1 activity caused by various genetic defects leading to lower locally available concentrations of cortisol (with or without significant changes of cortisol concentrations in the circulation) alter the hypothalamic-pituitary-adrenal (HPA) axis towards hyperandrogenism [6, 21]. This implies that presumably all experimental approaches using systemic manipulation of 11βHSD1 activity (both, transgenic and pharmacological) may trigger interfering systemic responses, i.e. dysregulation of the HPA axis and alterations of the ratio of glucocorticoids versus adrenal androgens (fig. 2). Adrenal androgens themselves and their metabolites are important modulators of inflammation in RA, as reviewed previously [22].

From transgenic animal studies, much less evidence exists concerning the role of 11βHSD2 in arthritis. No clear effects were seen in the initial studies [18]. More recently, transgenic overexpression of 11βHSD2 in osteoblasts was used to reduce the local glucocorticoid signaling. Indeed, it inhibited bone loss in the inflammatory model of K/BxN mouse serum-induced arthritis that usually leads to bone resorption, as demonstrated in the wild-type controls [23]. Moreover, this cell type-restricted alteration of glucocorticoid interconversion reduced local inflammatory activity, most likely via changes in the local levels of pro- and/or anti-inflammatory cytokines.

Taken together, notwithstanding the conclusiveness transgenic animal approaches can provide, results with these models alone cannot at present clarify the exact roles of the two 11βHSDs in arthritis synovial cells. There obviously is a need for more mouse models with cell type-specific knock-out (or overexpression) of 11βHSDs to delineate clearly the effects of each isoenzyme on glucocorticoid signaling in individual cell types and the systemic implications thereof – via paracrine or (neuro)endocrine (feedback) mechanisms [21, 24].

Studies Involving Synovial Cells and Related Specific Cell Types

In recent years, a solid body of evidence from more 'classical' experimental approaches appeared for the elucidation of 11βHSD-mediated modulation of glucocorticoid signaling in synovial cells. Three types of cell preparations are used in most of the functional studies mentioned: (1) tissue explants, homogenates or freshly isolated mixed synovial cells – which may best represent the in vivo mRNA expression, enzyme activities or metabolite concentrations, but lack resolution as to the cell types responsible; (2) cells propagated in vitro from synovial cell preparations – mostly synovial fibroblasts, which can be expanded and cultured for a long time, or (3) cell types that are found in RA synovial tissue but are more easily accessible from other sources, e.g. from blood or bone, etc.

As with the animal studies, more knowledge has accumulated concerning the function of 11βHSD1 than 11βHSD2. Cooper et al. [25] found in an osteosarcoma cell line and in primary osteoblasts that interleukin (IL)-1β or tumor necrosis factor (TNF)-α induced 11βHSD1 gene expression and activity, which increased glucocorticoid sensitivity of the cells. Expression of 11βHSD1 in tissue sec-

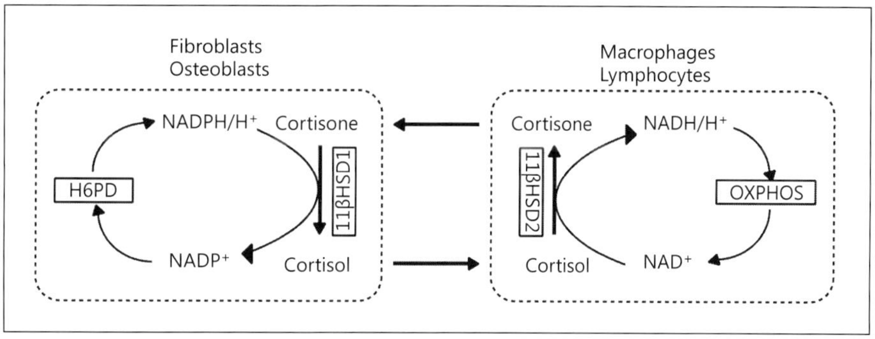

Fig. 3. Energy transfer by synovial glucocorticoid metabolism. 11βHSD2-expressing cells can generate NADH/H^+ from oxidation of cortisol, which can be further used in oxidative phosphorylation (OXPHOS) to provide ATP. Glucocorticoids are the diffusible intermediates. 11βHSD1 regenerates cortisol using NADPH/H^+, which is generated by the essential enzyme hexose-6-phosphate dehydrogenase (H6PD).

tions from patients with osteoarthritis (OA) and RA was found in the lining and sublining area by immunohistochemistry, and 11βHSD1 expression co-localized with the macrophage marker CD163 in double immunofluorescence [26]. Indeed, 11βHSD1 is induced in human monocytes upon differentiation to macrophages [27]. 11βHSD1 expression was induced by the anti-inflammatory IL-10 in synovial macrophages from control patients, but not in macrophages from RA patients [28]. In addition, CD163– cells, typically activated macrophages, but not CD3+ lymphocytes or prolyl 4-hydroxylase-positive fibroblasts, expressed 11βHSD1 [26]. However, the enzyme is also expressed in CD90+ fibroblasts from OA and RA patients [29], which might suggest that there are two subpopulations of synovial fibroblasts. In this study, IL-1β or TNF-α induced expression of 11βHSD1 and re-activation of cortisone by 11βHSD1 inhibited IL-6 production. Glucocorticoids also induce expression of 11βHSD1 and act synergistically with IL-1β or TNF-α in synovial fibroblasts and osteoblasts [30]. Cytokine-mediated induction of 11βHSD1 involves NF-κB signaling [31] and is necessary for secretion of a Wnt-antagonist by synovial fibroblasts [32].

Together with the cytokine signaling inhibitor studies in rats [20] and the knock-out mice work [19], a picture emerges in which initiation of inflammation by IL-1β/TNF-α prepares (sensitizes) synovial fibroblasts via expression of 11βHSD1 for the anti-inflammatory activity of glucocorticoids. This should contribute to resolution of local inflammation [4].

11βHSD2 entered the field of RA quietly, as it was found to be among 9 genes (from 4,300 analyzed) that were upregulated in peripheral blood mononuclear cells from patients with recent-onset RA at least 3-fold compared to healthy individuals [33]. In synovial tissue of patients with RA and OA who underwent knee replacement surgery, we found expression of 11βHSD2 in CD163+ macrophages and CD163– cells by double immunofluorescence labelling [26]. In this study, the ratio of cells positive for 11βHSD2 versus cells positive for 11βHSD1 was higher in RA than in OA, and biochemical analysis had shown that in RA the reactivation of cortisone to cortisol is impaired.

A subsequent study using samples from various anatomical sites indicated 11βHSD2 expression in synovial macrophages but a net reduction of cortisone [34]. An additional cell type of interest was found to express 11βHSD2: in lymphoblastoid B cell lines from RA-discordant twins, 11βHSD2 was the second most overexpressed gene in RA cases. Protein expression in synovial tissue of patients was correlated significantly with an inflammation score, suggesting a link between expression of 11βHSD2 and the degree of inflammation [35]. Interestingly, a similar link was also found for 11βHSD1 activity and levels of erythrocyte sedimentation rate [34].

The Inflamed Synovium – A Place for Two 11βHSDs

Thus, both 11βHSDs seem to be upregulated in RA (and possibly even in OA, when compared to non-inflamed tissue), albeit in different cell types. 11βHSD1 is most prominent in fibroblasts and osteoblasts, whereas 11βHSD2 is more prominent in macrophages and B cells (fig. 2). 11βHSD2 is not found in mouse macrophages during acute inflammation [36]. It is not expressed during differentiation of isolated human monocytes to macrophages, but it is found in the THP-1 macrophage cell line [27], consistent with the finding of an association of 11βHSD2 with cell proliferation [17]. In addition, 11βHSD2 expression was downregulated in osteoblasts upon treatment with IL-1β or TNF-α [25]. In combination, available experimental data suggest that 11βHSD2 is expressed: (1) in chronic inflammation, (2) in cells from the leukocyte lineage and (3) in cells that presumably seek to avoid glucocorticoid-induced apoptosis (fig. 2). The last appears to be quite reasonable, as glucocorticoids induce apoptosis in monocytes and macrophages, etc., but prevent apoptosis in other cells, such as fibroblasts [37].

However, there might be another pathway by which 11βHSD2 and glucocorticoids could provide an advantage to a cell surrounded by a growing fibroblast population: 11βHSD2 would allow a cell to tap the biosynthetic/energy resources of adjacent cells based on the shuttling of the diffusible glucocorticoids. Fibroblasts (or osteoblasts) reduce cortisone to cortisol, a reaction driven by their fuels. On the other side, a cortisol-avoiding macrophage or lymphocyte will inactivate cortisol in order to avoid apoptosis and gain some additional $NADH/H^+$, which can be further used in oxidative phosphorylation to provide ATP (fig. 3). That would provide a small but almost effortless energy income for macrophages/lymphocytes at the expense of fibroblasts.

Conclusions

The characteristics of the 11βHSDs explain the tightrope walk of glucocorticoid therapy for RA and, possibly, other chronic inflammatory diseases. Inhibition of 11βHSD1 may protect bone at the price of hindering resolution of inflammation. Inhibition of 11βHSD2 is accompanied by mineralocorticoid-like side effects, as does application of glucocorticoids in high doses. However, dosage should be high enough to hit the sensitive cells (and/or started before the 11βHSD2 even starts working in the synovial tissue). Combination therapies with biologicals (anti-IL-1β or anti-TNF) should reduce the side effects on bone. Either a targeted delivery system or a tool for cell type-specific inhibition of 11βHSD2 expression seems necessary to affect macrophages and lymphocytes optimally.

References

1 Hench PS, Kendall EC, Slocumb CH, Polley HF: The effect of a hormone of the adrenal cortex (17-hydroxy-11-dehydrocorticosterone; compound E) and of pituitary adrenocorticotropic hormone on rheumatoid arthritis. Proc Staff Meet Mayo Clin 1949;24:181–197.
2 Bailey E, Greaves MS, Murphy D, West HF: Corticosteroid metabolism and rheumatoid arthritis. Ann Rheum Dis 1966;25:516–524.
3 Murphy D, West HF: Catabolism and interconversion of cortisol and cortisone in human synovial tissue in vitro. Ann Rheum Dis 1969;28:637–643.
4 Hillier SG: Diamonds are forever: the cortisone legacy. J Endocrinol 2007;195:1–6.
5 Miller WL: Steroidogenic enzymes. Endocr Dev 2008;13:1–18.
6 Gathercole LL, Lavery GG, Morgan SA, Cooper MS, Sinclair AJ, Tomlinson JW, Stewart PM: 11β-Hydroxysteroid dehydrogenase 1: translational and therapeutic aspects. Endocr Rev 2013;34:525–555.
7 Chapman K, Holmes M, Seckl J: 11β-Hydroxysteroid dehydrogenases: intracellular gatekeepers of tissue glucocorticoid action. Physiol Rev 2013;93:1139–1206.
8 Seckl JR, Walker BR: 11β-Hydroxysteroid dehydrogenase type 1 as a modulator of glucocorticoid action: from metabolism to memory. Trends Endocrinol Metab 2004;15:418–424.
9 Tomlinson JW, Walker EA, Bujalska IJ, Draper N, Lavery GG, Cooper MS, Hewison M, Stewart PM: 11β-Hydroxysteroid dehydrogenase type 1: a tissue-specific regulator of glucocorticoid response. Endocr Rev 2004;25:831–866.
10 Albiston AL, Obeyesekere VR, Smith RE, Krozowski ZS: Cloning and tissue distribution of the human 11 β-hydroxysteroid dehydrogenase type 2 enzyme. Mol Cell Endocrinol 1994;105:R11–R17.
11 White PC, Agarwal AK, Nunez BS, Giacchetti G, Mantero F, Stewart PM: Genotype-phenotype correlations of mutations and polymorphisms in HSD11B2, the gene encoding the kidney isozyme of 11β-hydroxysteroid dehydrogenase. Endocr Res 2000;26:771–780.
12 Morris DJ, Latif SA, Hardy MP, Brem AS: Endogenous inhibitors (GALFs) of 11β-hydroxysteroid dehydrogenase isoforms 1 and 2: derivatives of adrenally produced corticosterone and cortisol. J Steroid Biochem Mol Biol 2007;104:161–168.
13 Balazs Z, Nashev LG, Chandsawangbhuwana C, Baker ME, Odermatt A: Hexose-6-phosphate dehydrogenase modulates the effect of inhibitors and alternative substrates of 11β-hydroxysteroid dehydrogenase 1. Mol Cell Endocrinol 2009;301:117–122.
14 Mitic T, Shave S, Semjonous N, McNae I, Cobice DF, Lavery GG, Webster SP, Hadoke PW, Walker BR, Andrew R: 11β-Hydroxysteroid dehydrogenase type 1 contributes to the balance between 7-keto- and 7-hydroxy-oxysterols in vivo. Biochem Pharmacol 2013;86:146–153.
15 Odermatt A, Kratschmar DV: Tissue-specific modulation of mineralocorticoid receptor function by 11β-hydroxysteroid dehydrogenases: an overview. Mol Cell Endocrinol 2012;350:168–186.
16 Condon J, Gosden C, Gardener D, Nickson P, Hewison M, Howie AJ, Stewart PM: Expression of type 2 11β-hydroxysteroid dehydrogenase and corticosteroid hormone receptors in early human fetal life. J Clin Endocrinol Metab 1998;83:4490–4497.
17 Rabbitt EH, Ayuk J, Boelaert K, Sheppard MC, Hewison M, Stewart PM, Gittoes NJ: Abnormal expression of 11β-hydroxysteroid dehydrogenase type 2 in human pituitary adenomas: a prereceptor determinant of pituitary cell proliferation. Oncogene 2003;22:1663–1667.
18 Holmes MC, Kotelevtsev Y, Mullins JJ, Seckl JR: Phenotypic analysis of mice bearing targeted deletions of 11β-hydroxysteroid dehydrogenases 1 and 2 genes. Mol Cell Endocrinol 2001;171:15–20.
19 Coutinho AE, Gray M, Brownstein DG, Salter DM, Sawatzky DA, Clay S, Gilmour JS, Seckl JR, Savill JS, Chapman KE: 11β-Hydroxysteroid dehydrogenase type 1, but not type 2, deficiency worsens acute inflammation and experimental arthritis in mice. Endocrinology 2012;153:234–240.
20 Ergang P, Leden P, Vagnerova K, Klusonova P, Miksik I, Jurcovicova J, Kment M, Pacha J: Local metabolism of glucocorticoids and its role in rat adjuvant arthritis. Mol Cell Endocrinol 2010;323:155–160.
21 Cooper MS, Stewart PM: 11β-Hydroxysteroid dehydrogenase type 1 and its role in the hypothalamus-pituitary-adrenal axis, metabolic syndrome, and inflammation. J Clin Endocrinol Metab 2009;94:4645–4654.
22 Schmidt M, Naumann H, Weidler C, Schellenberg M, Anders S, Straub RH: Inflammation and sex hormone metabolism. Ann NY Acad Sci 2006;1069:236–246.

23 Buttgereit F, Zhou H, Kalak R, Gaber T, Spies CM, Huscher D, Straub RH, Modzelewski J, Dunstan CR, Seibel MJ: Transgenic disruption of glucocorticoid signaling in mature osteoblasts and osteocytes attenuates K/BxN mouse serum-induced arthritis in vivo. Arthritis Rheum 2009;60:1998–2007.
24 Edwards C: Sixty years after Hench: corticosteroids and chronic inflammatory disease. J Clin Endocrinol Metab 2012;97:1443–1451.
25 Cooper MS, Bujalska I, Rabbitt E, Walker EA, Bland R, Sheppard MC, Hewison M, Stewart PM: Modulation of 11β-hydroxysteroid dehydrogenase isozymes by proinflammatory cytokines in osteoblasts: an autocrine switch from glucocorticoid inactivation to activation. J Bone Miner Res 2001;16:1037–1044.
26 Schmidt M, Weidler C, Naumann H, Anders S, Scholmerich J, Straub RH: Reduced capacity for the reactivation of glucocorticoids in rheumatoid arthritis synovial cells: possible role of the sympathetic nervous system? Arthritis Rheum 2005;52:1711–1720.
27 Thieringer R, Le Grand CB, Carbin L, Cai TQ, Wong B, Wright SD, Hermanowski-Vosatka A: 11β-hydroxysteroid dehydrogenase type 1 is induced in human monocytes upon differentiation to macrophages. J Immunol 2001; 167:30–35.
28 Antoniv TT, Ivashkiv LB: Dysregulation of interleukin-10-dependent gene expression in rheumatoid arthritis synovial macrophages. Arthritis Rheum 2006;54:2711–2721.
29 Hardy RS, Filer A, Cooper MS, Parsonage G, Raza K, Hardie DL, Rabbitt EH, Stewart PM, Buckley CD, Hewison M: Differential expression, function and response to inflammatory stimuli of 11β-hydroxysteroid dehydrogenase type 1 in human fibroblasts: a mechanism for tissue-specific regulation of inflammation. Arthritis Res Ther 2006;8:R108.
30 Kaur K, Hardy R, Ahasan MM, Eijken M, van Leeuwen JP, Filer A, Thomas AM, Raza K, Buckley CD, Stewart PM, Rabbitt EH, Hewison M, Cooper MS: Synergistic induction of local glucocorticoid generation by inflammatory cytokines and glucocorticoids: implications for inflammation-associated bone loss. Ann Rheum Dis 2010;69:1185–1190.
31 Ahasan MM, Hardy R, Jones C, Kaur K, Nanus D, Juarez M, Morgan SA, Hassan-Smith Z, Benezech C, Caamano JH, Hewison M, Lavery G, Rabbitt EH, Clark AR, Filer A, Buckley CD, Raza K, Stewart PM, Cooper MS: Inflammatory regulation of glucocorticoid metabolism in mesenchymal stromal cells. Arthritis Rheum 2012;64:2404–2413.
32 Hardy R, Juarez M, Naylor A, Tu J, Rabbitt EH, Filer A, Stewart PM, Buckley CD, Raza K, Cooper MS: Synovial DKK1 expression is regulated by local glucocorticoid metabolism in inflammatory arthritis. Arthritis Res Ther 2012;14:R226.
33 Olsen N, Sokka T, Seehorn CL, Kraft B, Maas K, Moore J, Aune TM: A gene expression signature for recent onset rheumatoid arthritis in peripheral blood mononuclear cells. Ann Rheum Dis 2004;63:1387–1392.
34 Hardy R, Rabbitt EH, Filer A, Emery P, Hewison M, Stewart PM, Gittoes NJ, Buckley CD, Raza K, Cooper MS: Local and systemic glucocorticoid metabolism in inflammatory arthritis. Ann Rheum Dis 2008;67:1204–1210.
35 Haas CS, Creighton CJ, Pi X, Maine I, Koch AE, Haines GK, Ling S, Chinnaiyan AM, Holoshitz J: Identification of genes modulated in rheumatoid arthritis using complementary DNA microarray analysis of lymphoblastoid B cell lines from disease-discordant monozygotic twins. Arthritis Rheum 2006;54:2047–2060.
36 Chapman KE, Coutinho A, Gray M, Gilmour JS, Savill JS, Seckl JR: Local amplification of glucocorticoids by 11β-hydroxysteroid dehydrogenase type 1 and its role in the inflammatory response. Ann NY Acad Sci 2006;1088: 265–273.
37 Viegas LR, Hoijman E, Beato M, Pecci A: Mechanisms involved in tissue-specific apoptosis regulated by glucocorticoids. J Steroid Biochem Mol Biol 2008;109:273–278.

NeuroImmunoModulation

Neuroimmunomodulation 2015;22:46–50
DOI: 10.1159/000362734

Published online: September 12, 2014

Clinical Trials Documenting the Efficacy of Low-Dose Glucocorticoids in Rheumatoid Arthritis

Theodore Pincus[a] Maurizio Cutolo[b]

[a]Rush University, Medical Center, Chicago, Ill., USA; [b]Research Laboratory and Academic Division of Clinical Rheumatology, Department of Internal Medicine, University of Genoa, Genoa, Italy

Key Words
Low-dose prednisone · Rheumatoid arthritis · Prednisolone · Randomized clinical trials

Abstract
Twelve clinical trials have documented that prednisone or prednisolone in doses of 10 mg/day or less is efficacious to improve function, maintain status and/or slow radiographic progression in patients with rheumatoid arthritis (RA). An early trial reported by de Andrade et al. [Ann Rheum Dis 1964; 23:158–162] in 1964 indicated that 5 mg of prednisolone at night was preferred to 5 mg of prednisone in the morning. Harris et al. [J Rheumatol 1983;10:713–721] documented the efficacy of 5 mg/day of prednisone in a non-double-blind trial in 1983. Two important trials in the 1990s by Kirwan [N Engl J Med 1995;333:142–146] using 7.5 mg/day, and the COBRA study by Boers et al. [Lancet 1997;350:309–318] with step-down from 60 mg rapidly tapered to 5 mg/day led to strong advocacy of low-dose glucocorticoids. In 2002, the first Utrecht Study [Ann Intern Med 2002;136:1–12] indicated that 10 mg/day prednisone slowed radiographic progression, a finding confirmed and extended in 2005 by Svensson et al. [Arthritis Rheum 2005;52:3360–3370] with 7.5 mg/day, and Wassenberg et al. [Arthritis Rheum 2005;52:3371–3380] with 5 mg/day of prednisolone. In 2008, Buttgereit et al. [Lancet 2008;371:205–214] reported CAPRA-1, which documented that modified-release prednisone or prednisolone taken at bedtime led to lower morning stiffness and IL-6 levels compared to usual morning prednisone. In 2009, Pincus et al. [Ann Rheum Dis 2009;68:1715–1720] reported a withdrawal clinical trial, in which patients who took 3 mg/day were gradually withdrawn to placebo, and dropped out at a significantly higher rate than control patients who were 'withdrawn' to prednisone. In 2012, a second Utrecht Study [Ann Intern Med 2012;156:329–339], CAMERA-II, documented that 10 mg of prednisone added to a 'treat-to-target' strategy with methotrexate provided incremental slowing of radiographic progression. An Italian study of patients with early RA who received step-up disease-modifying antirheumatic drug therapy over 2 years plus prednisolone or not indicated higher rates of clinical remission and sustained remission associated with 7.5 mg/day of prednisolone [Arthritis Res Ther 2012; 14:R112]. The CAPRA-2 trial [Ann Rheum Dis 2013;72:204–210] documented that modified-release nighttime prednisone or prednisolone was significantly more efficacious than placebo. Taken together, these 12 clinical trials indicate that low-dose glucocorticoids prednisone or prednisolone provides symptomatic relief, improved functional status and slowing of radiographic progression for patients with RA.

KARGER

E-Mail karger@karger.com
www.karger.com/nim

1021–7401/14/0222–0046$39.50/0

Theodore Pincus, MD
Rush University
Medical Center
Chicago, IL 60612 (USA)
E-Mail tedpincus@gmail.com

Introduction

The introduction of glucocorticoids for treatment of rheumatoid arthritis (RA) in 1948 by Hench et al. [1] did not require randomized control clinical trials, which were first conducted only in the 1940s [2, 3]. Documentation of dramatic clinical responses in a report published in 1949 [1] was sufficient to allow glucocorticoids to be available for prescription by physicians. The 1950 Nobel Prize in Physiology and Medicine was awarded to Hench, Kendall and Reichstein for the discovery and clinical application of glucocorticoids [4].

The efficacy of glucocorticoids was obvious from the first administration. However, the absence of formal clinical trials left a void concerning both optimal dosage and adverse events. Of note, the Mayo Clinic group that discovered glucocorticoids recommended in 1955 that doses equivalent to 5–10 mg/day of prednisone be used in the treatment of RA [5]. However, a dose of 20 mg/day of prednisolone was used in clinical trials in 1960 (after glucocorticoids were available for treatment) to compare with aspirin [6, 7]. While disease-modifying properties were documented in patients with RA [6, 7], the 'conventional wisdom' at that time (and, to a large extent, at this time) was that low doses were not 'disease modifying', i.e. did not slow radiographic progression.

Physicians tended to prescribe doses of glucocorticoids higher than 10 mg/day, or even 20 mg/day, and many adverse events were seen in many patients after taking these high doses over more than a few months [8]. Although the efficacy of parenteral and intra-articular glucocorticoids was recognized for particular clinical situations, a poor risk/benefit ratio was widely acknowledged for high-dose oral glucocorticoids because of long-term adverse events [8]. Therefore, by the late 1950s, oral glucocorticoids were regarded as appropriate in RA only for severe, potentially life-threatening situations or as short-term 'bridging therapy', while awaiting results of what were regarded as 'remission-inducing' disease-modifying antirheumatic drugs, such as parenteral gold therapy [8, 9] (the long-term effectiveness of which was greatly exaggerated [10]).

An Early Clinical Trial of Prednisolone 5 mg/Day

The first clinical trial involving low-dose glucocorticoids was reported by de Andrade et al. [9] of the Oxford Regional Rheumatism Research Center, Stoke Mandeville Hospital, Aylesbury, UK. This report will be discussed in some detail, as it is not well known and appears to provide important lessons not only about glucocorticoids but also about how knowledge is disseminated in clinical medicine. These investigators reported using low-dose glucocorticoids in routine clinical care [9], on the basis of recommendations by the Mayo Clinic group to use doses equivalent to 5–10 mg/day of prednisone [5]. They stated that their clinical practice of treating all patients with 7.5 mg/day or less was also based on 'observations made in the course of studying the phenomenon of morning stiffness' [9].

The clinical trial included 56 patients, all of whom were reported never to have received doses higher than 5 mg of prednisolone (in the early 1960s!). The investigators compared preferences for 5 mg/day of prednisolone as an evening dose versus a 5-mg morning dose, giving a placebo in the reciprocal pattern in a cross-over design. Overall, 28 of the 56 (50%) patients preferred the evening dose, only 2 the morning dose, 18 were inconsistent, 1 had no preference and 7 did not have suitable data for analysis due to a limited understanding of the trial [9]. The conclusion was that 5 mg of prednisolone at night was more efficacious than in the morning for the management of most RA patients [9].

The report noted that most patients in a clinical trial as well as in usual care experienced 'few severe adverse effects throughout the treatment of prednisolone in daily doses of 5–7.5 mg. The mild adverse effects, notably, bruising, seem[ed] to be related to duration of treatment' [9]. The prevalence of adverse events was substantially lower in patients who received <10 mg compared to 10 mg or more, after 25 weeks, at 25–50 weeks and, most strikingly, after 50 weeks of treatment. Prolongation of therapy 'rarely produced fresh adverse effects, though the incidence of purpura and bruising continued to increase. ... Pituitary adrenocortical reserve was found to be present in all of ten patients who had taken 5 mg prednisolone daily for up to 3.5 years' [9]. The authors concluded that 'our present policy is not to exceed a daily total of 7.5 mg in any but the most exceptional circumstances' [9].

The report also concluded that 'it would be surprising if so low a dose could retard deterioration in the joints, assessed radiographically'. As noted, this inference was consistent with the 'conventional wisdom', i.e. the prevailing paradigm at the time. However, that idea likely is incorrect, in view of recent data from subsequent clinical trials documenting that doses of 10 mg/day or less, including two trials of 5 mg/day [11, 12], slow radiographic progression [11–17]. Furthermore, a cohort of patients treated over indefinite periods by the authors (T.P.), in-

Table 1. Clinical trials documenting the value of low-dose prednisone in RA [10–17, 19–22]

First author	Reference	Dose, mg/day	Outcome(s)
de Andrade	[9]	5	Morning stiffness
Harris	[11]	5	Function, X-ray
Kirwan	[13]	7.5	X-ray
Boers (COBRA Trial)	[14]	60→5	ACR criteria, X-ray
van Everdingen	[15]	10	Tender joint count, X-ray
Svensson	[16]	7.5	X-ray
Wassenberg	[12]	5	X-ray
Buttgereit (CAPRA-1)	[19]	5 (modified release)	Morning stiffness
Pincus	[20]	≤5	Discontinuation of prednisone or placebo
Bakker	[17]	10	X-ray
Montecucco	[21]	12.5→7.5	Remission
Buttgereit (CAPRA-2)	[22]	5 (modified release)	ACR20, 50

cluding all seen in 2000, 80% with prednisone at doses less than 5 mg/day, had Larsen radiographic scores that were only 3% of maximum, far lower than expected [18].

It is not possible to attribute the slowing of radiographic progression entirely to prednisone, since almost all patients were also treated with methotrexate. However, this low level of radiographic progression is rarely seen only with long-term methotrexate monotherapy. Thus, it appears a possible consideration that doses as low as 3 mg/day of prednisone not only provide symptomatic relief [18], but can also slow radiographic progression, though this has not been documented in a formal clinical trial.

In retrospect, it appears that the assumption widely held in the 1960s that low-dose prednisone was unlikely to slow radiographic progression may have been unfortunate. Certainly, it appears to have deterred further development of these doses over 20–30 years. Until 19 years after the report by de Andrade et al. [9], no clinical trials involving low-dose prednisone were reported [11].

Clinical Trials of Low-Dose Prednisone during the 1980s and 1990s

Over the last 3 decades, 11 additional clinical trials have been conducted to document the efficacy of low-dose glucocorticoids in RA [11–17, 19–22] (table 1). Documentation of efficacy is summarized briefly in this article; documentation of safety in these clinical trials is summarized in the article by Da Silva in this special issue, p. 57.

Interest in low-dose glucocorticoids was given impetus by observations during the mid-1980s of severe functional declines [23, 24], radiographic progression [25], premature mortality [23] and frequent work disability [26] in patients with RA. These observations suggested that adverse effects associated with glucocorticoid therapy might be justified on the basis of severity of RA. For example, the use of glucocorticoids, even in doses of 60 mg/day, for treatment of malignant diseases is generally accepted by doctors and patients, although severe RA was shown to have a 5-year survival comparable to stage 4 Hodgkin's disease [27].

In 1983, a 24-week open non-blinded clinical trial of 5 mg/day of prednisone was reported with positive results to maintain functional status and slow radiographic progression in the prednisone versus control group [11]. This clinical trial began the modern era of low-dose prednisone treatment. A greater risk/benefit ratio of low-dose glucocorticoid therapy compared to high-dose glucocorticoids was reported, including disease-modifying properties with 5 mg/day of prednisone, now confirmed in 6 further clinical trials with different designs and endpoints [12–17], although only 5 mg/day of prednisone was used in only one other clinical trial [12].

Two important clinical trials of low-dose glucocorticoids were reported in the 1990s. Kirwan [13] reported significant slowing of radiographic progression over 2 years in patients treated with 7.5 mg/day of prednisolone compared to placebo. Landewé et al. [28] reported on the longterm statistical benefits of the COBRA study [see the article by Rasch et al. in this special issue; pp. 51–56], which began with 60 mg of prednisolone, rapidly tapered to 5 mg/day, as well as sulfasalazine and methotrexate, compared to sulfasalazine. Again, significant slowing of radiographic progression was seen, which was maintained years later after discontinuation of prednisolone.

The two senior investigators, Dr. Kirwan and Dr. Boers, became strong advocates of common use of low-dose glucocorticoids in patients with RA.

Clinical Trials of Low-Dose Prednisone since 2000

Since 2000, 8 clinical trials have documented significant benefits of low-dose glucocorticoids [12, 15–17, 19–22]. The first Utrecht Study compared 10 mg of prednisolone to placebo with benefits documented for joint count and slowing of radiographic progression [15]. Svensson et al. [16] performed the Barfot Study in which 7.5 mg of prednisolone was shown to retard radiographic progression. A similar study by Wassenberg et al. [12], published simultaneously in *Arthritis and Rheumatism*, indicated slowing of radiographic progression with 5 mg/day of prednisolone.

The CAPRA-1 (Circadian Administration of Prednisone in Rheumatoid Arthritis) clinical trial [19] showed substantial differences in morning stiffness, as well as in IL-6 levels, associated with 12 weeks of modified-release prednisone, compared to immediate-release prednisone taken in the conventional morning dose. There was no significant difference in other efficacy measures, and the safety profile did not differ between the two treatment groups [19].

A withdrawal clinical trial of patients taking 5 mg/day or less was conducted to recognize whether patients might have clinical efficacy at this low dose [20]. This clinical trial was based on long-term therapy using 3 mg of prednisone as the initial dose in 83% of patients treated in this clinical setting after 2000, compared to 10.6 mg/day in 1980–1985, 20 years earlier [29]. Only 31 patients volunteered for this clinical trial, as many patients refused to participate since they had already tried to taper and discontinue prednisone on several occasions, at the advice of other physicians and family, but were convinced that prednisone was helpful. Among participants, the rate of withdrawal was significantly higher in patients who had been gradually tapered to placebo compared to those who remained on identical prednisone tablets in doses less than 5 mg/day [20].

Since the endpoint was withdrawal from therapy, there was no attempt to judge effects on maintaining functional status or slowing radiographic progression [20]. However, analyses of patients treated over a 25-year period [29] and of 150 patients treated by the author in the year 2000 [30] revealed Larsen scores that were only 3% of maximum. These data strongly suggest slowing of radiographic progression, although that cannot be isolated definitively, since most patients also were treated with methotrexate and/or other disease-modifying antirheumatic drugs.

In 2012, a second Utrecht Study, CAMERA-II, documented that 10 mg of prednisone, added to a 'treat-to-target' strategy with methotrexate, provided incremental slowing of radiographic progression [16]. A second clinical trial involving modified-release prednisone, CAPRA-2, indicated that addition of modified-release prednisone to existing DMARD treatment led to higher ACR20 and ACR50 responses compared to placebo, and with similar adverse events in both groups, establishing that modified-release prednisone is superior to placebo treatment [22].

Conclusions

Taken together, these studies document that low-dose prednisone or prednisolone provide both symptomatic relief with improved functional status and slowing of radiographic progression. Low doses are also associated with few adverse events and prednisone doses of 5 mg or less/day do not affect the hypothalamic-pituitary-adrenal axis [30, 31].

Randomized controlled clinical trials are the optimal method to analyze the efficacy and adverse effects of low-dose glucocorticoids, but have many limitations, particularly in chronic diseases – including a short time frame, inflexible dosage schedules and patient selection – which inevitably limit the application of results in actual clinical care [32–34]. Furthermore, it is extremely difficult or impossible to study the adverse effects of glucocorticoids adequately over fewer than 5 years. Therefore, clinical trials require supplementation with observational data, as discussed in another article in this special issue (see Pincus et al., p. 89). Knowledge of the risk/benefit ratio of low-dose glucocorticoids over long periods requires both clinical trials as well as long-term observational studies.

References

1 Hench PS, Kendall EC, Slocumb CH, Polley HF: The effect of a hormone of the adrenal cortex (17-hydroxy-11-dehydrocorticosterone; compound E) and of the pituitary adrenocorticotropic hormone on rheumatoid arthritis. Proc Staff Meet Mayo Clin 1949;24:181.

2 Streptomycin treatment of pulmonary tuberculosis: a Medical Research Council investigation. Br Med J 1948;2:769–782.

3 Hill AB: Suspended judgment: memories of the British streptomycin trial in tuberculosis – the first randomized clinical trial. Controlled Clin Trials 1990;11:77–79.
4 Hench PS: The reversibility of certain rheumatic and non-rheumatic conditions by the use of cortisone or of the pituitary adrenocorticotropic hormone. Ann Intern Med 1952; 36:1–38.
5 Polley HF, Slocumb CH, Ward LE, Hench PS: Recognition and treatment of patients with chronic hypercortisonism. Ann Rheum Dis 1955;14:416–417.
6 Empire Rheumatism Council: Multi-centre controlled trial comparing cortisone acetate and acetyl salicylic acid in the long-term treatment of rheumatoid arthritis: results up to one year. Ann Rheum Dis 1955;14:353–367.
7 Empire Rheumatism Council: Multi-centre controlled trial comparing cortisone acetate and acetyl salicylic acid in the long-term treatment of rheumatoid arthritis: results of three years treatment. Ann Rheum Dis 1957;16: 277–289.
8 Benedek TG: History of the development of corticosteroid therapy. Clin Exp Rheumatol 2011;29(5 suppl 68):5–12.
9 de Andrade JR, McCormick JN, Hill AGS: Small doses of prednisolone in the management of rheumatoid arthritis. Ann Rheum Dis 1964;23:158–162.
10 Wolfe F, Hawley DJ: Remission in rheumatoid arthritis. J Rheumatol 1985;12:245–252.
11 Harris ED Jr, Emkey RD, Nichols JE, Newberg A: Low dose prednisone therapy in rheumatoid arthritis: a double blind study. J Rheumatol 1983;10:713–721.
12 Wassenberg S, Rau R, Steinfeld P, Zeidler H: Very low-dose prednisolone in early rheumatoid arthritis retards radiographic progression over two years: a multicenter, double-blind, placebo-controlled trial. Arthritis Rheum 2005;52:3371–3380.
13 Kirwan JR: The effects of glucocorticoids on joint destruction in rheumatoid arthritis. N Engl J Med 1995;333:142–146.
14 Boers M, Verhoeven AC, Markusse HM, van de Laar MAFJ, Westhovens R, van Denderen JC, et al: Randomised comparison of combined step-down prednisolone, methotrexate and sulphasalazine with sulphasalazine alone in early rheumatoid arthritis. Lancet 1997; 350:309–318.
15 van Everdingen AA, Jacobs JWG, van Reesema DRS, Bijlsma JWJ: Low-dose prednisone therapy for patients with early active rheumatoid arthritis: clinical efficacy, disease-modifying properties, and side effects. Ann Intern Med 2002;136:1–12.
16 Svensson B, Boonen A, Albertsson K, van der Heijde D, Keller C, Hafstrom I: Low-dose prednisolone in addition to the initial disease-modifying antirheumatic drug in patients with early active rheumatoid arthritis reduces joint destruction and increases the remission rate: a two-year randomized trial. Arthritis Rheum 2005;52:3360–3370.
17 Bakker MF, Jacobs JW, Welsing PM, Verstappen SM, Tekstra J, Ton E, et al: Low-dose prednisone inclusion in a methotrexate-based, tight control strategy for early rheumatoid arthritis: a randomized trial. Ann Intern Med 2012;156:329–339.
18 Pincus T, Sokka T, Castrejón I, Cutolo M: Decline of mean initial prednisone dosage from 10.3 to 3.6 mg/day to treat rheumatoid arthritis between 1980 and 2004 in one clinical setting, with long-term effectiveness of dosages less than 5 mg/day. Arthritis Care Res 2013; 65:729–736.
19 Buttgereit F, Doering G, Schaeffler A, Witte S, Sierakowski S, Gromnica-Ihle E, et al: Efficacy of modified-release versus standard prednisone to reduce duration of morning stiffness of the joints in rheumatoid arthritis (CAPRA-1): a double-blind, randomised controlled trial. Lancet 2008;371:205–214.
20 Pincus T, Swearingen CJ, Luta G, Sokka T: Efficacy of prednisone 1–4 mg/day in patients with rheumatoid arthritis: a randomised, double-blind, placebo controlled withdrawal clinical trial. Ann Rheum Dis 2009;68:1715–1720.
21 Montecucco C, Todoerti M, Sakellariou G, Scire CA, Caporali R: Low-dose oral prednisone improves clinical and ultrasonographic remission rates in early rheumatoid arthritis: results of a 12-month open-label randomised study. Arthritis Res Ther 2012;14:R112.
22 Buttgereit F, Mehta D, Kirwan J, Szechinski J, Boers M, Alten RE, et al: Low-dose prednisone chronotherapy for rheumatoid arthritis: a randomised clinical trial (CAPRA-2). Ann Rheum Dis 2013;72:204–210.
23 Pincus T, Callahan LF, Sale WG, Brooks AL, Payne LE, Vaughn WK: Severe functional declines, work disability, and increased mortality in seventy-five rheumatoid arthritis patients studied over nine years. Arthritis Rheum 1984;27:864–872.
24 Rasker JJ, Cosh JA: The natural history of rheumatoid arthritis: a fifteen year follow-up study. The prognostic significance of features noted in the first year. Clin Rheumatol 1984; 3:11–20.
25 Scott DL, Grindulis KA, Struthers GR, Coulton BL, Popert AJ, Bacon PA: Progression of radiological changes in rheumatoid arthritis. Ann Rheum Dis 1984;43:8–17.
26 Yelin E, Meenan R, Nevitt M, Epstein W: Work disability in rheumatoid arthritis: effects of disease, social, and work factors. Ann Intern Med 1980;93:551–556.
27 Pincus T, Brooks RH, Callahan LF: Prediction of long-term mortality in patients with rheumatoid arthritis according to simple questionnaire and joint count measures. Ann Intern Med 1994;120:26–34.
28 Landewé RB, Boers M, Verhoeven AC, Westhovens R, van De Laar MA, Markusse HM, et al: COBRA combination therapy in patients with early rheumatoid arthritis: long-term structural benefits of a brief intervention. Arthritis Rheum 2002;46:347–356.
29 Pincus T, Castrejon I, Sokka T: Long-term prednisone in doses of less than 5 mg/day for treatment of rheumatoid arthritis: personal experience over 25 years. Clin Exp Rheumatol 2011;29(5 suppl 68):S130–S138.
30 Pincus T, Sokka T, Kautiainen H: Patients seen for standard rheumatoid arthritis care have significantly better articular, radiographic, laboratory, and functional status in 2000 than in 1985. Arthritis Rheum 2005;52: 1009–1019.
31 Pincus T, Bijlsma JW, Braun J, Buttgereit F, Cutolo M: Low-dose glucocorticoids in rheumatic diseases: introduction. Clin Exp Rheumatol 2011;29(5 suppl 68):S2–S4.
32 Feinstein AR: An additional basic science for clinical medicine. II. The limitations of randomized trials. Ann Intern Med 1983;99:544–550.
33 Kaptchuk TJ: The double-blind, randomized, placebo-controlled trial: gold standard or golden calf? J Clin Epidemiol 2001;54:541–549.
34 Pincus T, Sokka T: Clinical trials in rheumatic diseases: designs and limitations. Rheum Dis Clin North Am 2004;30:701–724.

NeuroImmunoModulation

Neuroimmunomodulation 2015;22:51–56
DOI: 10.1159/000362728

Published online: September 12, 2014

Initial High-Dose Prednisolone Combination Therapy Using COBRA and COBRA-Light in Early Rheumatoid Arthritis

Linda A. Rasch[a] Lilian H.D. van Tuyl[a] Willem F. Lems[a] Maarten Boers[a, b]

Departments of [a]Rheumatology and [b]Epidemiology and Biostatistics, VU University Medical Center, Amsterdam, The Netherlands

Key Words

Combination drug therapy · Glucocorticoids · Rheumatoid arthritis · Clinical trial · Scholarly review

Abstract

Treatment with initial high-dose prednisolone and a combination of methotrexate (MTX) and sulfasalazine (SSZ) according to the COBRA regimen (Dutch acronym for combinatietherapie bij reumatoide artritis, 'combination therapy for rheumatoid arthritis'), has repeatedly been demonstrated to be very effective in early rheumatoid arthritis (RA). COBRA combination therapy is superior to initial monotherapy of SSZ and MTX, is also associated with a good long-term outcome, is as safe as other treatment regimes, and performs as well as the combination of high-dose MTX and the tumor necrosis factor antagonist infliximab. A pilot study with an intensified version of the COBRA combination therapy showed that strict monitoring and aggressive treatment intensification based on the Disease Activity Score can result in a remission rate of 90% in patients with active early RA. Also, the first results indicate that an attenuated variation on COBRA combination therapy, called 'COBRA-light', is effective in decreasing disease activity and is generally well tolerated. Based on these results, we conclude that initial high-dose prednisolone in combination with MTX and SSZ could or should be the first choice in early active RA since it is effective and safe, and the cost price of the drugs is low.

Introduction

Preferences for the initial treatment of early rheumatoid arthritis (RA) vary between rheumatologists, but disease-modifying antirheumatic drugs (DMARDs) and glucocorticoids (GC) are usually the first options, followed by tumor necrosis factor (TNF) antagonists for those patients who have incomplete responses on conventional DMARDs. Examples of conventional or synthetic DMARDs are, among others, methotrexate (MTX), sulfasalazine (SSZ) and hydroxychloroquine (HCQ). Recent recommendations of the European League against Rheumatism (EULAR) advise to start with MTX as early as possible after the diagnosis of RA, either alone or in combination with GC and/or other DMARDs. In case of failure, adverse events or incomplete responses, the patient is advised to start with a biological DMARD [1]. Initial treatment with high-dose prednisolone and a combination of DMARDs according to the COBRA trial (Dutch

KARGER

© 2014 S. Karger AG, Basel
1021–7401/14/0222–0051$39.50/0

E-Mail karger@karger.com
www.karger.com/nim

Linda A. Rasch
Department of Rheumatology, VU University Medical Center, Room ZH 3A-54
De Boelelaan 1117
NL–1081 HV Amsterdam (The Netherlands)
E-Mail l.rasch@vumc.nl

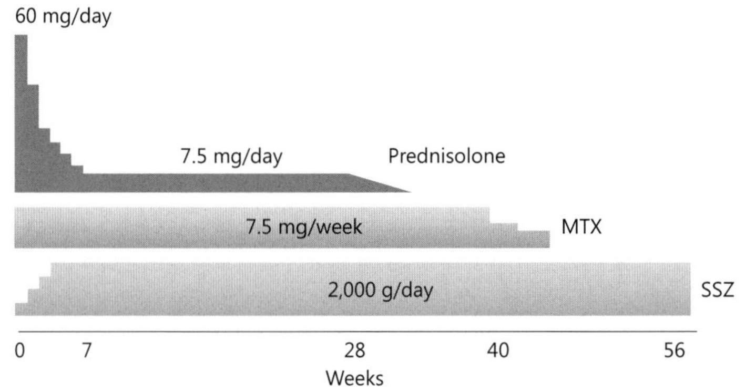

Color version available online

Fig. 1. Medication schedule of the original COBRA combination therapy.

acronym for combinatietherapie bij reumatoide artritis, 'combination therapy for rheumatoid arthritis', 1997) has repeatedly been demonstrated to be effective. In this review, we will discuss our experience with the different COBRA schedules.

COBRA Combination Therapy

The COBRA trial is the earliest study demonstrating the effect of treatment with a combination of DMARDs including initial high-dose GC [2]. The original COBRA trial was a 56-week multicenter, randomized controlled trial (RCT) among patients with recently diagnosed active RA (n = 156). For the first 28 weeks, all patients received 500 mg of SSZ per day, which was increased to 2,000 mg per day over a period of 3 weeks. In addition, the COBRA combination therapy arm was treated with a high dose of oral prednisolone of 60 mg per day, which was rapidly tapered to a low maintenance dose of 7.5 mg per day over 7 weeks, and 7.5 mg of MTX in a single stable weekly dose (table 1). From week 29 to 35, a day of zero prednisolone dose was introduced each week so that the prednisolone use was stopped after 36 weeks. MTX was tapered after 40 weeks of treatment (5 mg per week from week 40 to 42, 2.5 mg per week from week 43 to 45, and then stopped; see fig. 1). SSZ remained as the anchor drug after the other two drugs were withdrawn. The SSZ monotherapy arm, i.e. the control group, received matching placebos.

Within a few weeks, disease activity in both groups improved substantially, with a larger improvement in the COBRA combination therapy arm. Despite the low dose of prednisolone from week 7 to 28, the larger improvement of the COBRA combination therapy continued and a significant difference in Disease Activity Score (DAS) between both therapies was shown after 28 weeks (-2.1 ± 1.2 vs. -1.3 ± 1.2, $p < 0.0001$). However, after withdrawal of prednisolone and MTX, the difference between COBRA combination therapy and SSZ monotherapy decreased and was no longer significant after 56 weeks (-1.4 ± 1.2 and -1.3 ± 1.4, respectively), although a benefit in physical disability (Health Assessment Questionnaire) persisted. Radiographic damage was lower in the COBRA combination therapy arm than in the SSZ monotherapy arm up to week 80 ($p = 0.01$).

To investigate whether the benefits of the COBRA combination therapy were sustained over time, Landewé et al. [3] performed a 5-year follow-up study of patients in the COBRA trial. All patients were treated according to standard of care. Disease activity and functional ability were found to be similar and relatively stable over time in both groups. However, substantially less radiologic damage accrued in the COBRA arm: the mean change per year was 35% lower in COBRA compared to the SSZ group ($p = 0.03$).

Despite the effectiveness and positive 5-year follow-up results, rheumatologists remained concerned about the long-term effects of the initial high-dose of prednisolone, prompting a second follow-up study after 11 years [4]. This study found no differences in long-term outcome in functional capacity, disease activity and major co-morbidities between the two treatment groups. However, the benefits of COBRA on radiologic progression remained in evidence (and perhaps even continued to increase, depending on how one addresses selective drop-out).

Table 1. COBRA-like therapies for early active RA

	COBRA; Boers et al. [2]	COBRA/BeSt; Goekoop-Ruiterman et al. [5]	COBRA-plus; van Tuyl et al. [7]	COBRA-light; Den Uyl et al. [17]
Design	RCT, 56 weeks	RCT with blinded assessors, 2 years (up to 10 years of follow-up)	Randomized double-blind pilot trial, 40 weeks	Open, non-inferiority RCT, 1 year
Popula-tion	156 patients with early active RA	508 patients with early active RA	21 patients with active early RA	164 patients with early active RA
Therapy	*Combination therapy group* – MTX: 7.5 mg/week – Prednisolone: 60 mg/day which was tapered in 7 weeks to 7.5 mg/day, according to the following schedule: 60 mg/day in week 1 40 mg/day in week 2 25 mg/day in week 3 20 mg/day in week 4 15 mg/day in week 5 10 mg/day in week 6 7.5 mg/day in week 7 and thereafter – SSZ: 500 mg/day increased to 2,000 mg/day over a period of 3 weeks *Control group* – SSZ – Placebo for prednisolone and MTX	1. Monotherapy, started with MTX 2. Step-up combination therapy, started with MTX 3. Initial combination therapy, designed according to COBRA therapy, started with: – MTX: 7.5 mg/week – Prednisolone: 60 mg/day which was tapered in 7 weeks to 7.5 mg/day – SSZ: 2,000 mg/day – When the target was not met, treatment was followed subsequently by: intensification of MTX to 25–30 mg/week; MTX with cyclosporine and prednisolone; MTX with infliximab; leflunomide; gold with methylprednisolone; azathioprine with prednisolone 4. Initial combination therapy with MTX and infliximab	All patients were treated identically, with a modified COBRA scheme comprising HCQ – MTX: 10 mg/week – Prednisolone: 60 mg/day which was tapered in 7 weeks to 7.5 mg/day, according to the following schedule: 60 mg/day in week 1 40 mg/day in week 2 30 mg/day in week 3 20 mg/day in week 4 15 mg/day in week 5 10 mg/day in week 6 7.5 mg/day in week 7 and thereafter – SSZ: 2,000 mg/day – HCQ: 400 mg/day When the target was not met at week 8, MTX was intensified to 25 mg/week in 2 weeks; if still not met at week 21, infliximab was offered; if the target was met at week 8 but not at week 21, MTX was intensified.	*COBRA therapy group* – MTX: 7.5 mg/week – Prednisolone: 60 mg/day tapered to 7.5 mg/day in 6 weeks – SSZ: 1,000 mg/day, increased to 2,000 mg/day after 1 week *COBRA-light therapy group* – Prednisolone: 30 mg/day tapered to 7.5 mg/day in week 9, according to the following schedule: 30 mg/day in week 1 20 mg/day in week 2 15 mg/day in week 3 10 mg/day from week 4 to 8 7.5 mg/day from week 9 to 28 – MTX: 10 mg/week increased to 25 mg/week in week 9, according to the following schedule: 10 mg/week from week 2 to 4 17.5 mg/week from week 5 to 8 25 mg/week from week 9 to 26
Treatment goal/target	–	DAS44 ≤2.4	DAS or CTX (DAS28 ≤3.2 or CTX-II ≤150 ng/mmol creatinine)	Minimal disease activity (DAS44 <1.6)

BeSt = Behandel Strategiën; COBRA = Combinatietherapie Bij Reumatoide Artritis; CTX-II = C-terminal cross linking of type-II collagen; DAS = Disease Activity Score; HCQ = hydroxychloroquine; MTX = methotrexate; RA = rheumatoid arthritis; RCT = randomised controlled trial; SSZ = sulfasalazine.

COBRA/BeSt

Among the various therapeutic modalities, evidence for the clinical effectiveness of the original COBRA schedule was gradually accumulating. For this reason, COBRA combination therapy was included in the BeSt study (Dutch acronym for behandel strategiën, 'treatment strategies') in 2000 [5]. The BeSt study was a multicenter, RCT in which the clinical and radiographic outcomes of four different treatment strategies were compared: sequential monotherapy (group 1), step-up combination therapy (group 2), initial combination therapy with tapered high-dose prednisolone or COBRA therapy (group 3), and initial combination therapy with the TNF antagonist infliximab (group 4).

In contrast to the original COBRA combination therapy, the BeSt study used subsequent steps for patients whose medication failed. For patients assigned to group 3 (COBRA combination therapy), MTX was increased to 25–30 mg per week in case the target of DAS44 <2.4 was not met. The results of the BeSt study demonstrated that the arms with the initial combination therapy including either initial high-dose prednisolone (group 3, COBRA combination therapy) or infliximab (group 4) performed equivalently, resulting in earlier functional improvement and lower progression of radiographic joint damage after 1 year, compared to sequential monotherapy (group 1) or step-up combination therapy (group 2). Recently presented results of the 10-year follow-up data [6] showed a continued benefit of treat-to-target therapy, with 15% of prolonged drug-free remission. However, the difference in radiologic damage progression between the original treatment groups was no longer found.

COBRA-CTX-II Pilot Study

A few years later, in 2004, a pilot COBRA-CTX-II strategy was tested [7]. Several studies showed the effectiveness of monitoring disease activity according to the treat-to-target principle [8–10]. Furthermore, data of the COBRA trial showed that urinary excretion of C-terminal cross-linking of type II collagen (CTX-II), a marker to measure the extent of bone and cartilage degradation, predicted radiological progression over 5 years of follow-up more effectively than rheumatoid factor, baseline damage or disease activity [11–13]. For the COBRA-CTX-II pilot, we hypothesized that CTX-II might be more useful as a monitor for treatment intensification than disease activity measured by the DAS.

In a small pilot study (n = 21), patients were randomized to one of two monitoring strategies based on either frequent measurement of DAS or of the excretion of CTX-II. Patients and physicians were kept blinded to the monitoring strategy. Both groups received the COBRA schedule to which 400 mg of HCQ per day was added. MTX was increased to 25 mg per week if the target of DAS28 ≤3.2 or CTX-II ≤150 ng/mmol creatinine was not met at 8 weeks (table 1), and infliximab could be added after 21 weeks. This intensive treatment strategy, in combination with strict monitoring, proved to be feasible and resulted in a unique response with 90% of patients reaching DAS28-remission (DAS28 <2.6) after 40 weeks.

COBRA Combination Therapy in Clinical Practice

Despite its effectiveness, the original COBRA combination therapy was not often prescribed in clinical practice. Therefore, barriers and facilitating factors of the COBRA prescription were investigated by van Tuyl et al. [14, 15]. To explore the reasons for the reluctance to prescribe COBRA combination therapy, a short survey was performed. This survey showed that, although rheumatologists were convinced of the effectiveness of the COBRA combination therapy, they did not intend to prescribe COBRA therapy to their patients. The main concerns were the complexity of the drug schedule, the high initial dosage of 60 mg of prednisolone per day, inclusion of SSZ in the treatment schedule, and the low dosage of 7.5 mg of MTX per week [14].

To further explore this reluctance, focus group discussions were organized with rheumatologists as well as patients. A large discordance was found between what patients actually feel about COBRA therapy (mostly positive) and what rheumatologists think they feel (mostly negative). Besides the concerns about their patients' possible negative reaction, rheumatologists also perceived practical problems in prescribing and explaining COBRA therapy and they felt uncomfortable prescribing high doses of prednisolone, while the patients did not indicate that they had problems with taking many pills if that would improve their disease so dramatically [15].

To address the perceived barriers towards use of COBRA in daily clinical practice, an implementation strategy was designed and pilot tested [16]. A patient information booklet was distributed, including visual aids to explain the therapy, clear tables on the intake of the different drugs, and pre-printed prescriptions to speed up the prescribing process. The English language website containing the patient information material as well as the scientific data on COBRA therapy is currently online at www.cobratherapy.nl.

COBRA-Light Therapy

To overcome the rheumatologists' objections to the original COBRA schedule, our next step was the introduction of the so-called 'COBRA-light' strategy, which was compared to the original COBRA in a randomized, open, multicenter trial [17]. Patients assigned to the COBRA-light therapy started with 30 mg of prednisolone per day tapered to 7.5 mg per day in 9 weeks, and 10 mg of MTX per week with stepwise increments to 25 mg per week in 9 weeks. As in the BeSt study, patients assigned to the COBRA therapy could increase their MTX dose if the target was not met at 13 or 26 weeks (table 1). The cumulative dose of prednisolone after 28 weeks was 2,380 mg for the original COBRA combination therapy and 1,855 mg for the COBRA-light therapy.

After 26 weeks, disease activity was measured to determine the next treatment step: either DAS44 <1.6 – taper prednisolone in weekly steps and stop at week 38, or DAS44 ≥1.6 – start with TNF-antagonist (after first increasing MTX to 25 mg per week in the COBRA combination therapy arm). Disease activity rapidly decreased in both groups. The change in DAS44 at 26 weeks was –2.50 (1.21) for COBRA combination therapy and –2.18 (1.10) for COBRA-light therapy (between-group difference was 0.33; 95% CI –0.003 to 0.68), with most of the effect already reached after 13 weeks.

No significant differences were found for functional ability and C-reactive protein levels, except for erythrocyte sedimentation rate, which was lower in the COBRA arm ($p = 0.003$). The proportion of patients reaching minimal disease activity (DAS44 <1.6) did not differ significantly between both groups: 49% COBRA combination therapy versus 41% COBRA-light therapy. These results suggest that COBRA-light therapy is a feasible alternative to the original COBRA combination therapy in the first 6 months of treatment, since both therapies effectively lower disease activity and are generally well tolerated. Results at 1 year will be reported soon.

Summary

COBRA combination therapy is superior to initial monotherapy of either SSZ or MTX, and equal to high-dose MTX and infliximab in early active RA. Additionally, it is as safe as the other treatment regimens, and it is also associated with a good long-term outcome. A pilot study suggests that further intensification may substantially increase response. Furthermore, initial results of our latest trial suggest that high-dose MTX combined with lower initial doses of prednisolone give results equivalent to the original COBRA strategy. These results strongly suggest that the combination of MTX and prednisolone in intermediate to high initial doses should be the treatment of choice in patients with early active RA.

References

1 Smolen JS, Landewe R, Breedveld FC, Buch M, Burmester G, Dougados M, Emery P, Gaujoux-Viala C, Gossec L, Nam J, Ramiro S, Winthrop K, De Wit M, Aletaha D, Betteridge N, Bijlsma JW, Boers M, Buttgereit F, Combe B, Cutolo M, Damjanov N, Hazes JM, Kouloumas M, Kvien TK, Mariette X, Pavelka K, van Riel PL, Rubbert-Roth A, Scholte-Voshaar M, Scott DL, Sokka-Isler T, Wong JB, Van der Heijde D: EULAR recommendations for the management of rheumatoid arthritis with synthetic and biological disease-modifying antirheumatic drugs: 2013 update. Ann Rheum Dis 2014;73:492–509.

2 Boers M, Verhoeven AC, Markusse HM, van de Laar MA, Westhovens R, van Denderen JC, van Zeben D, Dijkmans BA, Peeters AJ, Jacobs P, van den Brink HR, Schouten HJ, van der Heijde DM, Boonen A, van der Linden S: Randomised comparison of combined step-down prednisolone, methotrexate and sulphasalazine with sulphasalazine alone in early rheumatoid arthritis. Lancet 1997;350:309–318.

3 Landewé RBM, Boers M, Verhoeven AC, Westhovens R, van de Laar MAFJ, Markusse HM, Van Denderen JC, Westedt ML, Peeters AJ, Dijkmans BAC, Jacobs P, Boonen A, van der Heijde DMFM, van der Linden S: COBRA combination therapy in patients with early rheumatoid arthritis: long-term structural benefits of a brief intervention. Arthritis Rheum 2002;46:347–356.

4 van Tuyl LHD, Boers M, Lems WF, Landewe RB, Han H, van der Linden S, van de Laar M, Westhovens R, van Denderen JC, Westedt ML, Peeters AJ, Jacobs P, Huizinga TWJ, van de Brink H, Dijkmans BAC, Voskuyl AE: Survival, comorbidities and joint damage 11 years after the COBRA combination therapy trial in early rheumatoid arthritis. Ann Rheum Dis 2010;69:807–812.

5 Goekoop-Ruiterman YPM, De Vries-Bouwstra JK, Allaart CF, Van Zeben D, Kerstens PJSM, Hazes JMW, Zwinderman AH, Ronday HK, Han KH, Westedt ML, Gerards AH, Van Groenendael JHLM, Lems WF, Van Krugten MV, Breedveld FC, Dijkmans BAC: Clinical and radiographic outcomes of four different treatment strategies in patients with early rheumatoid arthritis (the BeSt study): a randomized, controlled trial. Arthritis Rheum 2005;52:3381–3390.

6 Akdemir G, van den Broek M, Dirven L, Goekoop RJ, Han KH, Van Oosterhout M, Kerstens PJSM, Lems WF, Huizinga TWJ, Allaart CF: 10 years of treat-to-target therapy in rheumatoid arthritis patients (the BeSt study): clinical and radiological outcomes. Arthritis Rheum 2013;65:S620.

7 van Tuyl LH, Lems WF, Voskuyl AE, Kerstens PJ, Garnero P, Dijkmans BA, Boers M: Tight control and intensified COBRA combination treatment in early rheumatoid arthritis: 90% remission in a pilot trial. Ann Rheum Dis 2008;67:1574–1577.

8 Rantalaiho V, Kautiainen H, Korpela M, Hannonen P, Kaipiainen-Seppanen O, Mottonen T, Kauppi M, Karjalainen A, Laiho K, Laasonen L, Hakola M, Peltomaa R, Leirisalo-Repo M: Targeted treatment with a combination of traditional DMARDs produces excellent clinical and radiographic long-term outcomes in early rheumatoid arthritis regardless of initial infliximab: the 5-year follow-up results of a randomised clinical trial, the NEO-RACo trial. Ann Rheum Dis 2013, Epub ahead of print.

9 Bakker MF, Jacobs JW, Welsing PM, Verstappen SM, Tekstra J, Ton E, Geurts MA, van der Werf JH, van Albada-Kuipers GA, Jahangier-de Veen ZN, Van der Veen MJ, Verhoef CM, Lafeber FP, Bijlsma JW: Low-dose prednisone inclusion in a methotrexate-based, tight control strategy for early rheumatoid arthritis: a randomized trial. Ann Intern Med 2012;156: 329–339.

10 van Dongen H, van Aken J, Lard LR, Visser K, Ronday HK, Hulsmans HM, Speyer I, Westedt ML, Peeters AJ, Allaart CF, Toes RE, Breedveld FC, Huizinga TW: Efficacy of methotrexate treatment in patients with probable rheumatoid arthritis: a double-blind, randomized, placebo-controlled trial. Arthritis Rheum 2007;56:1424–1432.

11 Garnero P, Landewé R, Boers M, Verhoeven A, van der Linden S, Christgau S, van der Heijde D, Boonen A, Geusens P: Association of baseline levels of markers of bone and cartilage degradation with long-term progression of joint damage in patients with early rheumatoid arthritis: the COBRA study. Arthritis Rheum 2002;46:2847–2856.

12 Landewé RB, Geusens P, Boers M, van der Heijde DM, Lems W, Te Koppele J, van der Linden SJ, Garnero P: Markers for type II collagen breakdown predict the effect of disease-modifying treatment on long-term radiographic progression in patients with rheumatoid arthritis. Arthritis Rheum 2004;50: 1390–1399.

13 Landewé RB, Geusens P, Van der Heijde DM, Boers M, Van der Linden SJ, Garnero P: Arthritis instantaneously causes collagen type I and type II degradation in patients with early rheumatoid arthritis: a longitudinal analysis. Ann Rheum Dis 2006;65:40–44.

14 van Tuyl LHD, Plass AM, Lems WF, Voskuyl AE, Dijkmans BAC, Boers M: Why are Dutch rheumatologists reluctant to use the COBRA treatment strategy in early rheumatoid arthritis? Ann Rheum Dis 2007;66:974–976.

15 van Tuyl LHD, Plass AMC, Lems WF, Voskuyl AE, Kerstens PJSM, Dijkmans BAC, Boers M: Discordant perspectives of rheumatologists and patients on COBRA combination therapy in rheumatoid arthritis. Rheumatology 2008;47:1571–1576.

16 van Tuyl LH, Plass AM, Lems WF, Voskuyl AE, Kerstens PJ, Dijkmans BA, Boers M: Facilitating the use of COBRA combination therapy in early rheumatoid arthritis: a pilot implementation study. J Rheumatol 2009;36: 1380–1386.

17 Den Uyl D, Ter Wee MM, Boers M, Kerstens P, Voskuyl A, Nurmohamed M, Raterman H, Van Schaardenburg D, Van Dillen N, Dijkmans B, Lems W: A non-inferiority trial of an attenuated combination strategy ('COBRA-light') compared to the original COBRA strategy: clinical results after 26 weeks. Ann Rheum Dis 2014;73:1071–1078.

NeuroImmunoModulation

Neuroimmunomodulation 2015;22:57–65
DOI: 10.1159/000362726

Published online: September 12, 2014

Safety of Glucocorticoids in Rheumatoid Arthritis: Evidence from Recent Clinical Trials

Tânia Santiago José António P. da Silva

Rheumatology Unit, Centro Hospitalar e Universistário de Coimbra, Faculdade de Medicina da Universidade de Coimbra, Coimbra, Portugal

Key Words
Rheumatoid arthritis · Glucocorticoids · Safety · Toxicity · Review · Randomized controlled trials

Abstract
Glucocorticoids are one of the most effective treatments for rheumatoid arthritis, with well-established efficacy in controlling the disease symptoms and structural progression. Fears regarding their toxicity are reflected in common recommendations for the use of the lowest possible dose for the shortest possible time. We herein review toxicity data obtained in randomized clinical trials of low-dose glucocorticoid in rheumatoid arthritis, given that observational studies cannot guarantee the avoidance of bias by indication. Seven eligible randomized controlled trials were identified. These publications do not identify any strong signal of relevant toxicity of glucocorticoid in doses of up to 10 mg of prednisone equivalent/day for up to 2 years. However, the quantity (1,100 patient years of exposure) and especially the quality of evidence are too limited to establish conclusions. A large prospective trial dedicated to the toxicity of low-dose glucocorticoid is dearly needed. Meanwhile, adherence to recommendations on standardized methodologies for the registration and report of glucocorticoid adverse events is essential to improve our knowledge and competence in the best management of these important medications.

Introduction

Despite being in use for six decades of intense medical progress, glucocorticoids (GCs) still have a pivotal role in the management of rheumatoid arthritis (RA), resisting persistent (and sometimes alarming) news about their toxicity. The recent accumulation of solid evidence supporting their ability to reduce radiographic progression and modify the disease course, even at low dose, has stressed the need for a balanced re-assessment of risks and benefits [1–3]. The concept that adverse events (AEs) are potentially serious and depend on the dose and duration of use support recommendations that the minimum dose should be used for the shortest possible time, always in combination with other disease-modifying anti-rheumatic drugs [4].

However, the evidence required on which to base such decisions remains very limited. Theoretical constructs about the potential direct toxicity of GCs must acknowledge their potential benefits derived from the systemic reduction of inflammation. Data derived from observational studies need to be critically appraised in terms of the risks of bias by indication and the effect of unaccounted confounders [5]. RA is, per se, associated with a higher risk of many AEs, which are also considered as side effects of GCs, such as cardiovascular disease, osteoporosis and fractures, and decreased insulin sensitivity

KARGER

E-Mail karger@karger.com
www.karger.com/nim

1021–7401/14/0222–0057$39.50/0

José António P. da Silva, MD, PhD
Head of Department, Serviço de Reumatologia
Centro Hospitalar Universitário de Coimbra
PT–3000-076 Coimbra (Portugal)
E-Mail jdasilva@huc.min-saude.pt

[6]. Patients with higher disease severity are more likely to be prescribed GCs and in higher dosages. Consequently, negative effects arising as a consequence of the disease per se and its co-morbidities may be attributed to the concomitant GC treatment. Disentangling such confounding issues cannot be achieved through observational studies. Valid and robust conclusions can only be obtained through properly designed prospective controlled trials.

A previous comprehensive review concluded that the evidence regarding many AEs of low-dose GCs remains elusive and that the risk/benefit balance of low-dose GC treatment deserves reassessment as it may differ significantly from that of medium- and high-dose treatment [7]. In this paper we update this review with the evidence from recent randomized controlled trials (RCTs) in RA on the safety of low- and medium-dose GC treatment lasting at least 12 months.

Materials and Methods

We performed a systematic literature search in MEDLINE databases, looking at clinical trial data and meta-analyses published between January 2005 and July 2013. Eligibility assessment was performed independently, on the basis of title and abstract, by the two authors. Disagreements were resolved by discussion.

Studies were included for further analysis if: (1) they were RCTs; (2) they included adult patients with RA; (3) they focused on exposure to systemic GC therapy (excluding intra-articular injections) in one arm and non-exposure in another, otherwise comparable, study arm; (4) GCs were used in dosages <30 mg of prednisone or equivalent per day; (5) they lasted 6 months or longer, and (6) they were published in English, French, Spanish, Italian or Portuguese. Studies that had already been included in the 2006 review were not subject to a detailed data search and analysis as the previous work had been done with access to the current study data [7].

Studies Included

The seven RCTs selected for inclusion in this review, together with their main features and findings, are presented in table 1 [8–15]. The first four [9–12] were already considered by Da Silva et al. [7] in 2006. In total 1,274 patients were included in these trials, 624 being exposed to low-dose GCs (5–10 mg of prednisone equivalent/day) for 2 years in 514 patients and 1 year in the remaining 110, totaling 1,138 patient years of GC exposure.

We excluded the BeSt, the COBRA and the CARDERA trials because: (1) high doses of prednisolone were used and/or (2) GC treatment was interrupted long before final evaluation and/or the complexity of the treatment schedule precluded clear attribution of side effects to GC use. Only patients with active early RA (<2 years) were included in these studies. The treatment groups were generally composed of disease-modifying anti-rheumatic drugs (DMARDs) with or without GCs. GC exposure was well defined in the included RCTs.

Findings from RCTs and Meta-Analysis

Overall Risk of AEs

A previous comprehensive review of the safety of low-dose GC treatment in RA published in 2006 [7] included raw data from four RCTs [8–12]. The authors did not perform a meta-analysis because they considered that the systems used for AE elicitation were too diverse to allow for an integrated evaluation.

Hoes et al. [5] conducted a meta-analysis of low- to medium-dose GCs used for at least 1 month in a variety of diseases and settings. They found that the reported GC-related AE rate was lower in RA studies (43/100 patient years) than in polymyalgia rheumatic (80/100 patient years) and, especially, inflammatory bowel disease (555/100 patient years). The rate of AEs depended on the study design and disease. Overall, the conclusions of this meta-analysis supported the modest toxicity profile of GCs in rheumatic diseases previously described [7].

Ravindran et al. [16] performed a meta-analysis on the safety of medium- to long-term GC therapy in RA. Six RCTs were included, four of which were also considered in the review of Da Silva et al. [7]. Based on the number of patients withdrawn due to AEs as a primary outcome for toxicity (OR = 1.09; 95% CI 0.52, 2.25), the toxicity of GC therapy in RA was described as 'limited'. Consideration of the number of AEs per patient year (OR = 1.19; 95% CI 0.91, 1.57) or the number of serious AEs (OR = 1.06; 95% CI 0.67, 1.67) produced similar results, which were not statistically different from placebo.

In both the Utrecht Study and CAMERA-II Study, the Utrecht group concludes that AEs with low- to medium-dose GCs were generally mild or even favorable [10–14] (table 1). Actually, in the 2-year CAMERA-II Study, a methotrexate-based tight control trial, fewer patients in the prednisolone (P) group experienced AEs or worse compared with the non-prednisolone (NoP) group.

Bone Loss and Fractures

Bone mineral density (BMD) was systematically assessed in four of the seven trials included in this review. None of these studies found statistically significant effects of prednisone upon BMD when compared with placebo (see table 1). Fracture incidences were small and similar between the groups, when reported [17]. However, in the Utrecht Study GC treatment was associated with a doubling of the incidence of radiological vertebral fractures, although this did not reach statistical significance [10].

It is important to emphasize that the individual trials we identified are too small and/or too short in duration

Table 1. Characteristics of the 7 RCTs of low- and medium-dose GC in RA included in this review

Study	Author and year	RA patients, n; RA duration at entry	P group, n	GC dose, mg/day	Study duration, months	Association DMARDs	Method of monitoring AEs	AEs reported	Results of AEs (P group vs. NoP group)
ARC	Kirwan [8], 1995; Hickling et al. [9], 1998	128 patients with active RA; <2 years	61	7.5	24	Free choice		Lumbar spine (% BMD loss in 11 P and 10 NoP patients over 2 years	2.96 (5.59) vs. 1.29 (4.64); not significant[1]
								Hip (% BMD loss in 11 P and 10 NoP patients over 2 years)	1.19 (3.16) vs. 4.02 (2.45), p = 0.04 at 2 years[1]
								New-onset diabetes	0 vs. 1 case
								Weight gain	'Both groups increased in weight, but there was no statistically significant mean increase in body weight in either group'
								Blood pressure	'there were no significant increases in blood pressure in either group'; 2 developed hypertension in the P group vs. 1 in the NoP group
UTRECHT	van Everdingen et al. [10], 2002	81 patients with early active RA; <1 year	40	10	24	SSZ rescue	Standardized lists was used to document AEs	Overall (withdrawals due to AEs)	0 vs. 0% ('no patients left the study because of adverse effects related to the study medication')
								New osteoporotic fractures	5 (12.5%) vs. 2 (4.9%)
								BMD lumbar spine (mean T score at baseline and at 2 years)	Changed from –0.8 (0.3) to –1.1 (0.3) in the P group and from –0.7 (0.3) to –0.6 (0.3) in the NoP group; not statistically significant intra- or intergroups[1]
								BMD femoral neck (mean T score at baseline and at 2 years)	Changed from –1.8 (0.2) to –1.9 (0.2) in the P group and from –1.9 (0.2) to –1.9 (0.2) in the NoP group; not statistically significant intra- or intergroups[1]
								Glycemia	In contrast to the placebo group, the mean serum glucose level (± SD) increased significantly in the P group, from 5.1 ± 0.6 mmol/l to 5.9 ± 1.9 mmol/l ($p < 0.01$)
								Newly developed hyperglycemia	Diabetes: 2 (5%) vs. 1 (2.4%)
								Mean weight gain (SD)	77 (19) to 80 (20) kg in the P group, p = 0.001, at 0 and 2 years, respectively; no statistically significant change in the placebo group
								Blood pressure	No difference
								Newly developed hypertension	7 (17.5%) vs. 6 (14.6%)
								Infections requiring antibiotics	17 (42.5%) vs. 22 (53.6%)
								Ophthalmological	Glaucoma: 1 (2.5%) vs. 0 Cataract: 1 (2.5%) vs. 1 (2.5%)
								Gastrointestinal	Peptic symptoms: 7 (17.5%) vs. 3 (7.3%) Ulcer bleeding: 1 (2.5%) vs. 2 (4.6%)
								Neuropsychological	Depression: 1 (2.5%) vs. 2 (4.6%)
								Dermatological	No difference

Table 1 (continued)

Study	Author and year	RA patients, n; RA duration at entry	P group, n	GC dose, mg/day	Study duration, months	Association DMARDs	Method of monitoring AEs	AEs reported	Results of AEs (P group vs. NoP group)
BARFOT	Svensson et al. [13], 2005	250 patients with early active RA; <1 year	119	7.5	24	MTX or SSZ	AE were registered at the follow-up visits and were either spontaneously reported or revealed by laboratory values	Overall (temporary or permanent withdrawal due to AEs)	26 vs. 24 (NS)
								BMD lumbar spine (mean BMD at baseline and at 2 years; n = 189)	1.14±0.16 and 1.11±0.16 in the P group vs. 1.17±0.21 and 1.16±0.21 in the NoP group; no significant difference
								BMD femoral neck (mean BMD at baseline and at 2 years; n = 189)	0.91±0.15 and 0.90±0.16 in the P group vs. 0.90±0.15 and 0.87±0.15 in the NoP group; no significant difference
								New cases of diabetes	1 (0.8%) vs. 0
								Weight gain as cause for withdrawal	1 vs. 1 case
								Infections	No infection leading to discontinuation in P group
CAMERA-II	Bakker et al. [14], 2012; van der Goes et al. [17], 2013	236 patients with early RA; <2 years	117	10	24	MTX	Standard list of AEs to be related with PDN, yearly DEXA	Overall (withdrawal due to AEs)	14 vs. 17%
								New onset diabetes mellitus	1 (0.8%) vs. 1 (0.8%)
								Glucose levels increased by >1.0 mmol/l at 2 years vs. baseline	13 patients (11%) P group vs. 9 patients (8%) in the NoP group
								Weight gain (variation weight between baseline and 2 years)	2.9 (4.2) vs. 1.3 (5.3) kg, p = 0.03
								Infections	Treated with antibiotics, 1 (0.85%) P group vs. 0 NoP group
								Ophthalmological	Glaucoma: 0 P group vs. 1 (0.8%) NoP group Cataract: 1 (0.9%) P group vs. 0
								Clinical osteoporotic fractures	1 vs. 0%
								Lumbar spine BMD (mean change at 2 years vs. baseline)	2.4 vs. 3.4%; 'significant differences between the treatment strategies in sBMD or the trend over time could not be demonstrated'
								Femoral neck BMD (change at 2 years vs. baseline)	'The sBMD in the left hip did not change significantly during the 2 years of treatment'
Montecucco	Montecucco et al. [15], 2012	220 patients with early RA; <1 year	110	6.25	12	MTX	Information not available	Overall	No data: '… few relevant side effects related to low-dose PDN medication'
								Osteoporotic fractures	No data: 'sample size and length of follow-up did not allow to measure the effect of GC on rare events'
								Hyperglycemia	2 (0.9%) P group vs. 0 (?)
								Gastrointestinal	Epigastric pain, 4 (1.8%) in the P group vs. 0 (?)

TC = Total cholesterol; MTX = methotrexate; SSZ = sulfasalazine; QCT = quantitative computed tomography; DEXA = dual-energy X-ray absorptiometry; PDN = prednisone.
[1] Derived from Da Silva et al. [7] 2006 (web-only additional material).

to allow definite conclusions regarding osteoporosis and fractures. Furthermore, in most studies, all participants were treated with calcium and vitamin D.

Lee et al. [18] conducted a meta-analysis to assess the negative effect of low-dose GC on BMD in RA patients. Seven studies with 353 patients and 343 controls were included. They concluded, from looking at BMD change from baseline, that 'corticosteroids have a clear effect on both lumbar and femoral BMDs (SMD [standardized mean difference] = –0.354, p = 0.009; SMD = –0.488, p = 0.024, respectively)'. The authors interpret the data as suggesting that low-dose corticosteroid treatment accelerates bone loss in patients with RA, which overcomes the potential benefit derived from disease control.

Other Musculoskeletal AEs

No cases of osteonecrosis or myopathy were reported in any of the reviewed trials.

Glucose Metabolism and Diabetes

Data from the seven extensively reviewed studies on GC in RA are quite reassuring in this respect: no relevant differences in the number of cases of new-onset diabetes were seen in either of the trials. The Utrecht Study found the least favorable results: a significant increase in mean (SD) fasting glucose was seen in the P group [from 5.1 (0.6) at baseline to 5.9 (1.9) mmol/l at 2 years, p < 0.01]. However, hyperglycemia, as defined by the World Health Organization, developed in only 2 patients in the P group (n = 40) and 1 in the NoP group (n = 41; table 1). On the other hand, in the CAMERA-II Study, performed by the same group, 10 mg of prednisone daily did not lead to higher glucose levels or an increased incidence of diabetes over 2 years of treatment [14].

The impact of GCs in glucose metabolism in RA was addressed in a very elegant study performed by Hoes et al. [19]. They measured glucose tolerance, insulin sensitivity and β-cell function in two RA populations (58 chronic GC users and 82 who were GC naïve) and in healthy controls, with no known type 2 diabetes mellitus. Chronic GC users and GC-naïve patients with RA presented similar metabolic parameters, with decreased insulin sensitivity and β-cell function in comparison to healthy controls. Cumulative doses of GCs had a negative impact on glucose tolerance state and insulin sensitivity. The results highlight a complex interplay of three factors: (1) the RA-induced pro-inflammatory state negatively impacts on glucose metabolism; (2) GC downregulates disease activity, which may diminish this effect, but (3) GC itself impairs glucose metabolism [20].

Weight Gain

Weight gain is one of the most frequently reported GC AEs [21]. Significantly more weight gain associated with GC therapy was reported in the Utrecht, LDPT and CAMERA-II studies, but not in the WOSERACT study (see table 1). In a sub-analysis of the CAMERA-II study, Jurgens et al. [22] attributed part of the difference in weight gain between the groups to an earlier and better control of disease activity with prednisone.

Cardiovascular Risk Factors and Atherosclerosis

A meta-analysis performed by Ruyssen-Witrand et al. [23] highlighted that an association between low-dose GCs (<10 mg/day of prednisone) and major cardiovascular events was found in four out of six trials. These events included: myocardial infection [HR = 1.7 (1.2–2.3)], stroke [OR = 4.36 (1.60–11.90)], cardiovascular mortality [HR = 2.03 (1.25–3.32)] and a composite index of cardiovascular events [in the group of rheumatoid factor-positive RA, HR = 2.21 (1.22–4.00)]. Two studies did not find any significant association between low-dose GC exposure and mortality [OR = 2.25 (0.29–102.5)] or a composite index of CV events [OR = 1.3 (0.8–2.0)].

Carotid atherosclerosis and endothelial function were assessed by ultrasonography in a subset of 67 patients from the BARFOT study, 5 years after the start of their first DMARD: 21 patients had been treated with 7.5 mg of prednisolone daily for 2 years and 13 continuously for 5 years before vascular evaluation, in comparison with 33 non-exposed patients [24]. The authors found that low-dose prednisolone did not influence endothelial function and atherosclerosis in RA (table 1) [25]. There were no significant differences in the levels of total cholesterol, high-density lipoprotein (HDL) and low-density lipoprotein (LDL) cholesterol, lipoprotein(a), triglycerides or homocysteine levels between those exposed and those not exposed to GC treatment.

Of the recent trials, WOSERACT is the only one [11] that refers to lipid levels. The conclusion sounds reassuring: 'There was no significant difference in the lipids at outset or at 2 years in those patients in whom it was measured (total cholesterol/HDL cholesterol)'. Unfortunately, no actual data is provided.

Of the three trials reporting on blood pressure, two (Utrecht and WOSERACT) found no significant variation in blood pressure induced by low-dose prednisolone. The LDPT trial reported that 6.5% of the patients treated with prednisolone developed new-onset hypertension during the study, in comparison with 2.2% of the controls (table 1).

Infections

None of the RCTs included in this review found an increased incidence of any kind of infections over the 1–2 years of follow-up (table 1). A recent systematic review [26] compiled data from 21 RCTs (including 1,026 GC-treated patients with RA) and 42 observational studies. The estimated relative risk (RR) of infection associated with GC therapy differed significantly between the RCTs [RR 0.97 (95% CI 0.69–1.36)] and the observational studies [RR 1.67 (95% CI 1.49–1.87)]. The GC dose, cumulative exposure, time-varying exposure, co-therapy, comorbidity, recruitment methods, outcome and bias (in particular publication bias) contributed to the significant heterogeneity observed in the observational studies [26, 27].

Dermatological AEs

The Utrecht Study included a regular dermatological check [10]. Non-infectious AEs were registered in 15% of the P group and 9.8% of the controls over 2 years. No cases of skin thinning or easy bruising were reported. Curiously, 5 episodes of erysipelas were observed in 4 patients, all from the control group. None of the other studies reported on skin manifestations.

Ophthalmological AEs

Only 3 of the 7 extensively reviewed trials on GC-related AEs in RA report on ocular AEs. According to the description of methodology, the LDPT seems to have adopted the most stringent ocular evaluation protocol: all participants have an eye examination at the start and at the end of 2 years [12]. Three new cases of glaucoma were identified in the P group (n = 93) during the 2 years of treatment as opposed to none in the control group (n = 96). The incidence of cataracts was of 5 and 6, respectively.

Gastrointestinal AEs

Four reports described gastrointestinal side effects (table 1). Peptic symptoms and ulcers appear to be more frequent in GC-treated patients, but the role of potential confounders, such as concomitant NSAIDs, are not clearly addressed. No cases of pancreatitis were reported.

Neuropsychological AEs

Only the Utrecht Study provides a report of neuropsychological disorders, which were regularly assessed and documented. There was no hint of a relevant impact of low prednisolone (10 mg per day) over 2 years [10].

Discussion

Overall, the toxicity profile of low-dose GCs described in these seven RCTs seems mild and hardly different from that described for placebo, except for weight gain and glaucoma. However, the evidence is scarce and of poor quality.

None of the available RCTs were designed to assess the toxicity of GCs and the attention dedicated to toxicity seems to be, in general, very limited. In CAMERA-II [14], a systematic register was made, based on a standard list of AEs 'known to be related to prednisone'. In most other cases, the methodology used to define and identify AEs is unclear or extremely diverse, thus clouding conclusions. Reporting is also highly variable and frequently poorly informative, for example, mean group levels of glucose do not inform how many participants have significant increases in glycemia or new-onset diabetes [28]. Potential confounders, such as concomitant therapies, are not systematically reported or accounted for. Overall, the studies have relatively small dimensions and a type II error cannot be excluded: the absence of statistical significance for observed numerical differences in the incidence of some side effects may be due to small sample sizes rather a true reflection of reality. We also need to recognize that the short duration of the available trials may hinder the identification of adverse effects related to long-term treatment.

The dosages of GCs used also deserve consideration. We have adopted the definition of low- and medium-dose GC as <7.5 mg and <30 mg of prednisone equivalent per day, respectively. This is consistent with previous recommendations [29]. However, it could be argued that the term low-dose should be restricted to regimes below 5 mg of prednisolone equivalent per day, on the basis that such dosages do not induce significant long-term adrenal suppression [30, 31].

Some authors also argued that the available clinical trials use higher GC doses than are really necessary to achieve the desired clinical results, thus contributing to unnecessary toxicity [32]. In a recent retrospective study, minimal long-term AEs were observed in patients who have taken a very low dose of GC for more than 10 years [33].

Certainly, the limitations of the available clinical trials need to be taken into account when analyzing the evidence: absence of evidence for serious toxicity is not the same as evidence that such toxicity is absent. However, the limitations of the alternative source of information – non-randomized observational studies – especially confounding by indication, cannot be ignored either. Whereas typical efficacy-driven clinical trials may artificially reduce the description of true toxicity, observational studies tend to have an equally erroneous and pernicious opposite effect, which cannot be totally overridden by statistical corrections.

Definite conclusions about the safety of GCs require randomized clinical trials with sufficient dimension and duration and with appropriate standardization in the definition and monitoring of AEs [34]. Such a trial will probably never happen at the hands of the pharmaceutical industry, but its need cannot be ignored by the clinical and scientific community. How can we continue to so frequently use medications we know so little about? Incredible as it may seem, the toxicity of low-dose GCs remains an orphan condition in rheumatology!

Meanwhile, it would be of great assistance if new trials adhered to standardized procedures for the monitoring and reporting of GC-related AEs, such as those recommended by the EULAR GC task force [28]. Research to improve the existing tools to measure some of these side effects (such as cutaneous and psychological side effects) is greatly needed.

In summary, on the basis of this literature review of the safety of low-to-medium doses of GCs in RA, including a careful review of seven RCTs, our main conclusion is that evidence to support clear conclusions regarding safety remains limited both in quantity and quality. In the last decade, more attention has been given to monitoring and reporting AEs in clinical trials, although scarce evidence was added to the comprehensive review of Da Silva et al. [7] published in 2006. Evidence-based recommendations for patient education, monitoring and prevention of GC-related AE in rheumatic diseases have been published [28, 34, 35]. Adherence to the standardized interventions and assessments conveyed in these documents may significantly contribute to our ability to reduce the GC-related AEs in RA and optimize their use for the benefit of patients.

References

1 Jacobs JW: Lessons for the use of non-biologic anchor treatments for rheumatoid arthritis in the era of biologic therapies. Rheumatology (Oxford) 2012;51(suppl 4):iv27–iv33.

2 Jacobs JW, van Everdingen AA, Verstappen SM, Bijlsma JW: Follow-up radiographic data on patients with rheumatoid arthritis who participated in a two-year trial of prednisone therapy or placebo. Arthritis Rheum 2006;54:1422–1428.

3 Kirwan JR, Bijlsma JW, Boers M, Shea BJ: Effects of glucocorticoids on radiological progression in rheumatoid arthritis. Cochrane Database Syst Rev 2007:CD006356.

4 Strand V, Simon LS: Low dose glucocorticoids in early rheumatoid arthritis. Clin Exp Rheumatol 2003;21:S186–S190.

5 Hoes JN, Jacobs JW, Verstappen SM, Bijlsma JW, Van der Heijden GJ: Adverse events of low- to medium-dose oral glucocorticoids in inflammatory diseases: a meta-analysis. Ann Rheum Dis 2009;68:1833–1838.

6 Wasko MC, Kay J, Hsia EC, Rahman MU: Diabetes mellitus and insulin resistance in patients with rheumatoid arthritis: risk reduction in a chronic inflammatory disease. Arthritis Care Res (Hoboken) 2011;63:512–521.

7 Da Silva JA, Jacobs JW, Kirwan JR, Boers M, Saag KG, Ines LB, de Koning EJ, Buttgereit F, Cutolo M, Capell H, Rau R, Bijlsma JW: Safety of low dose glucocorticoid treatment in rheumatoid arthritis: published evidence and prospective trial data. Ann Rheum Dis 2006;65:285–293.

8 Kirwan JR: The effect of glucocorticoids on joint destruction in rheumatoid arthritis: the arthritis and rheumatism council low-dose glucocorticoid study group. N Engl J Med 1995;333:142–146.

9 Hickling P, Jacoby RK, Kirwan JR, et al: Joint destruction after glucocorticoids are withdrawn in early rheumatoid arthritis. Br J Rheumatol 1998;37:930–936.

10 van Everdingen AA, Jacobs JW, Siewertsz van Reesema DR, Bijlsma JW: Low-dose prednisone therapy for patients with early active rheumatoid arthritis: clinical efficacy, disease-modifying properties, and side effects: a randomized, double-blind, placebo-controlled clinical trial. Ann Intern Med 2002;136:1–12.

11 Capell HA, Madhok R, Hunter JA, Porter D, Morrison E, Larkin J, Thomson EA, Hampson R, Poon FW: Lack of radiological and clinical benefit over two years of low dose prednisolone for rheumatoid arthritis: results of a randomised controlled trial. Ann Rheum Dis 2004;63:797–803.

12 Wassenberg S, Rau R, Steinfeld P, Zeidler H: Very low-dose prednisolone in early rheumatoid arthritis retards radiographic progression over two years: a multicenter, double-blind, placebo-controlled trial. Arthritis Rheum 2005;52:3371–3380.

13 Svensson B, Boonen A, Albertsson K, van der Heijde D, Keller C, Hafstrom I: Low-dose prednisolone in addition to the initial disease-modifying antirheumatic drug in patients with early active rheumatoid arthritis reduces joint destruction and increases the remission rate: a two-year randomized trial. Arthritis Rheum 2005;52:3360–3370.

14 Bakker MF, Jacobs JW, Welsing PM, Verstappen SM, Tekstra J, Ton E, Geurts MA, van der Werf JH, van Albada-Kuipers GA, Jahangier-de Veen ZN, van der Veen MJ, Verhoef CM, Lafeber FP, Bijlsma JW: Low-dose prednisone inclusion in a methotrexate-based, tight control strategy for early rheumatoid arthritis: a randomized trial. Ann Intern Med 2012;156:329–339.

15 Montecucco C, Todoerti M, Sakellariou G, Scire CA, Caporali R: Low-dose oral prednisone improves clinical and ultrasonographic remission rates in early rheumatoid arthritis: results of a 12-month open-label randomised study. Arthritis Res Ther 2012;14:R112.

16 Ravindran V, Rachapalli S, Choy EH: Safety of medium- to long-term glucocorticoid therapy in rheumatoid arthritis: a meta-analysis. Rheumatology (Oxford) 2009;48:807–811.

17 van der Goes MC, Jacobs JW, Jurgens MS, Bakker MF, van der Veen MJ, van der Werf JH, Welsing PM, Bijlsma JW: Are changes in bone mineral density different between groups of early rheumatoid arthritis patients treated according to a tight control strategy with or without prednisone if osteoporosis prophylaxis is applied? Osteoporos Int 2013;24:1429–1436.

18 Lee YH, Woo JH, Choi SJ, Ji JD, Song GG: Effects of low-dose corticosteroids on the bone mineral density of patients with rheumatoid arthritis: a meta-analysis. J Investig Med 2008; 56:1011–1018.
19 Hoes JN, van der Goes MC, van Raalte DH, van der Zijl NJ, den Uyl D, Lems WF, Lafeber FP, Jacobs JW, Welsing PM, Diamant M, Bijlsma JW: Glucose tolerance, insulin sensitivity and β-cell function in patients with rheumatoid arthritis treated with or without low-to-medium dose glucocorticoids. Ann Rheum Dis 2011;70:1887–1894.
20 Buttgereit F: Do the treatment with glucocorticoids and/or the disease itself drive the impairment in glucose metabolism in patients with rheumatoid arthritis? Ann Rheum Dis 2011;70:1881–1883.
21 Morrison E, Crosbie D, Capell HA: Attitude of rheumatoid arthritis patients to treatment with oral corticosteroids. Rheumatology (Oxford) 2003;42:1247–1250.
22 Jurgens MS, Jacobs JW, Geenen R, Bossema ER, Bakker MF, Bijlsma JW, van Albada-Kuipers IA, Ehrlich JC, Lafeber FP, Welsing PM: Increase of body mass index in a tight controlled methotrexate-based strategy with prednisone in early rheumatoid arthritis: side effect of the prednisone or better control of disease activity? Arthritis Care Res (Hoboken) 2013;65:88–93.
23 Ruyssen-Witrand A, Fautrel B, Saraux A, Le Loet X, Pham T: Cardiovascular risk induced by low-dose corticosteroids in rheumatoid arthritis: a systematic literature review. Joint Bone Spine 2011;78:23–30.
24 Hafstrom I, Rohani M, Deneberg S, Wornert M, Jogestrand T, Frostegard J: Effects of low-dose prednisolone on endothelial function, atherosclerosis, and traditional risk factors for atherosclerosis in patients with rheumatoid arthritis: a randomized study. J Rheumatol 2007;34:1810–1816.
25 Engvall IL, Svensson B, Tengstrand B, Brismar K, Hafstrom I: Impact of low-dose prednisolone on bone synthesis and resorption in early rheumatoid arthritis: experiences from a two-year randomized study. Arthritis Res Ther 2008;10:R128.
26 Dixon WG, Suissa S, Hudson M: The association between systemic glucocorticoid therapy and the risk of infection in patients with rheumatoid arthritis: systematic review and meta-analyses. Arthritis Res Ther 2011;13:R139.
27 Widdifield J, Bernatsky S, Paterson JM, Gunraj N, Thorne JC, Pope J, Cividino A, Bombardier C: Serious infections in a population-based cohort of 86,039 seniors with rheumatoid arthritis. Arthritis Care Res (Hoboken) 2013;65:353–361.
28 van der Goes MC, Jacobs JW, Boers M, Andrews T, Blom-Bakkers MA, Buttgereit F, Caeyers N, Cutolo M, Da Silva JA, Guillevin L, Kirwan JR, Rovensky J, Severijns G, Webber S, Westhovens R, Bijlsma JW: Monitoring adverse events of low-dose glucocorticoid therapy: EULAR recommendations for clinical trials and daily practice. Ann Rheum Dis 2010;69:1913–1919.
29 Buttgereit F, da Silva JA, Boers M, Burmester GR, Cutolo M, Jacobs J, Kirwan J, Kohler L, Van Riel P, Vischer T, Bijlsma JW: Standardised nomenclature for glucocorticoid dosages and glucocorticoid treatment regimens: current questions and tentative answers in rheumatology. Ann Rheum Dis 2002; 61:718–722.
30 Daly JR, Myles AB, Bacon PA, Beardwell CG, Savage O: Pituitary adrenal function during corticosteroid withdrawal in rheumatoid arthritis. Ann Rheum Dis 1967;26:18–25.
31 Barden N: Implication of the hypothalamic-pituitary-adrenal axis in the physiopathology of depression. J Psychiatry Neurosci 2004;29: 185–193.
32 Pincus T, Swearingen CJ, Luta G, Sokka T: Efficacy of prednisone 1–4 mg/day in patients with rheumatoid arthritis: a randomised, double-blind, placebo controlled withdrawal clinical trial. Ann Rheum Dis 2009;68:1715–1720.
33 Pincus T, Sokka T, Castrejon I, Cutolo M: Decline of mean initial prednisone dosage from 10.3 to 3.6 mg/day to treat rheumatoid arthritis between 1980 and 2004 in one clinical setting, with long-term effectiveness of dosages less than 5 mg/day. Arthritis Care Res (Hoboken) 2013;65:729–736.
34 Hoes JN, Jacobs JW, Boers M, Boumpas D, Buttgereit F, Caeyers N, Choy EH, Cutolo M, Da Silva JA, Esselens G, Guillevin L, Hafstrom I, Kirwan JR, Rovensky J, Russell A, Saag KG, Svensson B, Westhovens R, Zeidler H, Bijlsma JW: EULAR evidence-based recommendations on the management of systemic glucocorticoid therapy in rheumatic diseases. Ann Rheum Dis 2007;66:1560–1567.
35 Duru N, van der Goes MC, Jacobs JW, Andrews T, Boers M, Buttgereit F, Caeyers N, Cutolo M, Halliday S, Da Silva JA, Kirwan JR, Ray D, Rovensky J, Severijns G, Westhovens R, Bijlsma JW: EULAR evidence-based and consensus-based recommendations on the management of medium to high-dose glucocorticoid therapy in rheumatic diseases. Ann Rheum Dis 2013;72:1905–1913.

NeuroImmunoModulation

Neuroimmunomodulation 2015;22:66–71
DOI: 10.1159/000362729

Published online: September 12, 2014

Glucocorticoids in Early Rheumatoid Arthritis: Are the Benefits of Joint-Sparing Effects Offset by the Adverse Effect of Osteoporosis? The Effects on Bone in the Utrecht Study and the CAMERA-II Study

Johannes W.G. Jacobs   Johannes W.J. Bijlsma   Jacob M. van Laar

Department of Rheumatology and Clinical Immunology, University Medical Center Utrecht, Utrecht, The Netherlands

Key Words
Glucocorticoid · Rheumatoid arthritis · Prednisone · Radiological joint damage · Osteoporosis · Bone loss

Abstract
This paper reviews the clinical effects on bone of 10 mg of prednisone daily in early rheumatoid arthritis, given for 2 years in the Utrecht Study and in the second CAMERA (Computer-Assisted Management in Early Rheumatoid Arthritis) Study, and addresses the question whether there were joint-sparing effects and whether these were offset by adverse effects, especially osteoporosis. We conclude that a 2-year adjunct treatment with 10 mg of prednisone daily increases the benefits of disease-modifying antirheumatic drug therapy and has joint-sparing properties, even if added to the tight control methotrexate-based strategy aiming for remission. Importantly, with good control of inflammation and adequate use of calcium, vitamin D and bisphosphonates – according to national or international guidelines – steroid-induced osteoporosis is rare over 2 years.

Introduction

Glucocorticoids (GCs) are key drugs of therapeutic regimens in most inflammatory and autoimmune rheumatic conditions because of their effectiveness, versatility and low cost. Early data shortly after the introduction of GCs suggested potential slowing of radiographic progression in rheumatoid arthritis (RA) [1]. Nonetheless, because of adverse effects associated with high or moderate GC doses, for decades thereafter GCs were prescribed in RA primarily for their symptomatic effects. The Utrecht Study published in 2002 and the second CAMERA (Computer-Assisted Management in Early Rheumatoid Arthritis) Study published in 2012 also investigated the potential slowing of progression of radiographic joint damage by GCs in early RA [2, 3]. This paper reviews the clinical effects on bone found in these studies and addresses the question of whether there were joint-sparing effects and whether they were offset by adverse effects, especially osteoporosis.

KARGER

E-Mail karger@karger.com
www.karger.com/nim

1021–7401/14/0222–0066$39.50/0

J.W.G. Jacobs, MD, PhD
Department of Rheumatology and Clinical Immunology, F02.127
University Medical Center Utrecht, Box 85500
NL–3508 GA Utrecht (The Netherlands)
E-Mail j.w.g.jacobs@umcutrecht.nl

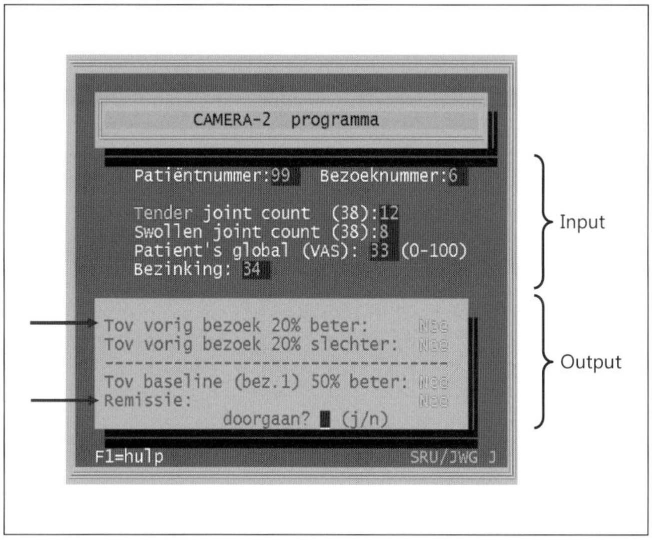

Fig. 1. The CAMERA studies Dutch computer decision program. In the input section, patient number ('Patiëntnummer'), visit number ('Bezoeknummer'), TJC assessing 38 joints, SJC assessing 38 joints, patient's global VAS and ESR ('Bezinking') are entered. In the output section, at the arrows, the result regarding >20% improvement compared to the previous visit 1 month earlier ('Tov vorig bezoek 20% beter') is given as yes ('ja') or no ('nee'), and whether there is remission ('Remissie') yes ('ja') or no ('nee'). Improvement >20% was defined as >20% improvement in SJC AND (Boolean) >20% improvement in ≥2 out of TJC, ESR and VAS. Remission was defined as SJC = 0 AND (Boolean) ≥2 out of TJC ≤3, VAS ≤20 mm and ESR ≤20 mm/h^{1st}. Protocolized strategy steps were based on these results (programmer: J.W.G.J.).

The Utrecht Study

This was a 2-year, double-blind, randomized, placebo-controlled clinical trial investigating the effect of medium-dose GCs as initial disease-modifying monotherapy in disease-modifying antirheumatic drug (DMARD)-naïve patients with early active RA [2]. Eighty-one patients were randomized to 10 mg of prednisone orally daily or placebo, next to a non-steroidal anti-inflammatory drug. After 6 months, sulfasalazine (2 g daily) could be added to the therapy if needed. The study was approved by the Ethical Committee, but nowadays it would be considered unethical to compare the effects of prednisone to those of placebo in patients who do not receive a DMARD for at least 6 months. Radiographs of hands and feet were taken at entry and every 6 months thereafter and scored with the Sharp-van der Heijde score [4].

The most important result of the study was that – from month 12 on – radiological scores showed less progression of joint damage in the prednisone-treated group compared to the placebo group, which was a statistically significant and clinically relevant finding. Nevertheless, progression of joint damage was still considerable in the prednisone-treated group too; mean (SD) changes in Sharp-van der Heijde scores from baseline at 2 years were 16 (23) and 29 (26) for the prednisone and placebo group, respectively. After the trial, prednisone was tapered and stopped, if possible. Radiographic scoring of hands and feet at about 3 years after the end of the Utrecht Study in available patients was performed according to the Sharp-van der Heijde method. Patients of the former prednisone group had significantly less progression compared to those of the former placebo group [5]. We concluded that the gain in slowing down of radiographic joint damage in patients with early active RA treated with prednisone was not lost after the end of prednisone treatment. This result is in line with follow-up results of the COBRA trial [6].

In the Utrecht Study, glucocorticoid-induced osteoporosis, i.e. vertebral fractures, occurred in 5 patients in the prednisone group (n = 40) versus 2 patients in the placebo group (n = 41; p = 0.26). Calcium had been supplemented in all patients, but nowadays generally more intensive preventive therapy is applied: calcium, vitamin D and a bisphosphonate. Other adverse effects were similar between both groups.

The Second CAMERA Study (CAMERA-II)

After the Utrecht Study, the first CAMERA Study was performed (see summary in box 1). From this first CAMERA Study, we concluded that a tight control strategy with methotrexate (MTX), aiming for remission (treat-to-target) in early RA with the help of a computer decision program (fig. 1), resulted in a better outcome over 2 years than a less tight MTX-strategy without a computer decision program [7]. See box 2 for a short explanation of the concepts of tight control and treat-to-target.

Based on the results of the Utrecht Study and the first CAMERA Study, the primary research question of CAMERA-II was whether prednisone would still have disease-modifying properties in early RA, as in the Utrecht Study, when added to a highly effective tight control MTX-based computer-assisted strategy aimed at remission, similar to that of the first of the CAMERA studies. CAMERA-II was a 2-year, prospective, randomized, placebo-controlled, double-blind, multicenter trial; all the included 236 patients with early RA (symptoms <1 year) were treated with an MTX-based tight control strategy and were randomly assigned to 10 mg of prednisone per day or placebo-prednisone [3].

Box 1. Summary of the first CAMERA Study [7, 22]

This was a 2-year population-based, randomized, open-label prospective multicenter treatment strategy trial among 299 early RA patients, who had a symptom duration of less than 1 year and were DMARD- and glucocorticoid-naïve. Patients were randomized to either a tight control MTX-based treatment strategy (n = 151), based on computer-guided monthly assessments of predefined response criteria, or to an at that time conventional MTX-based strategy (n = 148), based on regular clinical practice with 3-monthly visits. Both strategies were aiming at remission (treat to target).
For both strategies, data on SJC and TJC, both assessing 38 joints, ESR and VAS for global health were collected by the rheumatologist at every visit. In the tight control strategy these data were entered at each monthly visit into a computer decision program by the rheumatologist. The program calculated whether or not there was a >20% improvement (defined as >20% improvement in SJC and in ≥2 out of TJC, ESR and VAS), compared to the previous visit 1 month earlier, and whether or not there was remission (defined as SJC = 0 and ≥2 out of these 3 criteria: TJC ≤3, VAS ≤20 mm and ESR ≤20 mm/h^{1st}; see fig. 1). If neither a >20% improvement or remission was present, the strategy was intensified according to protocol. For the conventional strategy, dose adjustments were performed based on the opinion of the treating rheumatologist (mainly focused on the SJC) at each 3-monthly visit.
Both strategies started with oral MTX 7.5 mg/week, which could be stepped up in steps of 5 mg/week towards a maximum oral MTX dose of 30 mg/week. This was followed, if needed, by switching from oral to subcutaneous MTX and, as a next step, by adding cyclosporine to the MTX medication. If patients fulfilled the criteria for sustained remission, defined as remission for at least 3 months, MTX was reduced stepwise by 2.5 mg/week as long as patients met the remission criteria; otherwise the dose of MTX was continued or increased again according to protocol. At baseline and subsequently yearly, joint damage was assessed on radiographs of hands and feet.
In the tight control strategy group 76 (50%) patients achieved at least one period of sustained remission during the 2-year trial (the primary outcome), compared to 55 patients (37%) in the conventional strategy group (p = 0.03). Areas under the curve for nearly all clinical disease activity variables were significantly lower – that is, there was a better clinical effect – for the tight control strategy group compared with the conventional strategy group. In both strategy groups, approximately 50% of patients did not progress regarding radiological joint damage over the 2 years. For the other 50%, there was a trend toward less progression in the tight control strategy group compared to the conventional strategy group.
We concluded that tight control treatment with MTX, aiming for remission, resulted in a better outcome over 2 years and that the computerized decision program could be a helpful tool in daily clinical practice.

Box 2. The concepts of tight control and treat-to-target strategies

A tight control strategy in RA is a treatment strategy with frequent clinical checks and – if needed – dose and medication adjustments, tailored to the individual RA patient, to achieve within a certain limited period of time (in early RA preferentially within the 'window of opportunity') a level of low disease activity and, preferentially, remission.
A treat-to-target strategy in RA is a treatment strategy that aims at achieving, preferentially within a certain limited period of time, a predefined level of low disease activity and, preferentially, remission. This predefined treatment target is defined by clear criteria.
Although these 2 concepts are similar, they are not identical.

The starting dose of MTX was 10 mg/week orally; MTX treatment in both groups was tailored to the individual patient at monthly visits on the basis of predefined response criteria aiming for remission (treat-to-target principle), applying the same variables and the same computer decision program as used in the first CAMERA Study (box 1; fig. 1). At baseline and every 4 weeks thereafter, swollen joint count (SJC; 0–38 joints), tender joint count (TJC; 0–38 joints), erythrocyte sedimentation rate (ESR), and visual analogue scale (VAS; 0–100 mm; 100 mm worst) for general well-being were assessed. Treatment was intensified in cases where patients had not improved sufficiently (sufficient improvement defined as >20% improvement in SJC and in ≥2 variables of TJC, ESR and VAS) compared to the previous visit 1 month earlier, by increasing the MTX dosage stepwise, switching to subcutaneous therapy with methotrexate (scMTX) at maximal (tolerated) oral MTX dose and, as a next step if needed, adding cyclosporine treatment.

Shortly after the trial was started, the protocol was amended: adalimumab replaced cyclosporine as a last strategy step, to be added to the maximum dosage of scMTX (fig. 2). This amendment was based on our finding of lack of effect of the cyclosporine strategy step in the first CAMERA Study [8]. If sustained remission (defined as an SJC of 0 and at least 2 out of the following: TJC ≤3, VAS of well-being ≤20 mm, ESR ≤20 mm/h^{1st}, all for at least 3 months) was achieved, MTX was reduced gradually by 2.5 mg/week each month as long as remission was present, according to the principle of patient-tailored tight control. After the 2-year trial, prednisone was tapered and stopped, if possible.

Fig. 2. The CAMERA-II tight control step-up strategy. If >20% improvement or remission was not achieved, the strategy was intensified according to this scheme. If patients had remission for at least 3 months (sustained remission), MTX was reduced stepwise by 2.5 mg/week as long as patients met remission criteria; otherwise the dose of MTX was continued or increased again according to protocol. Prednisone was tapered at the end of the study and stopped, if possible.

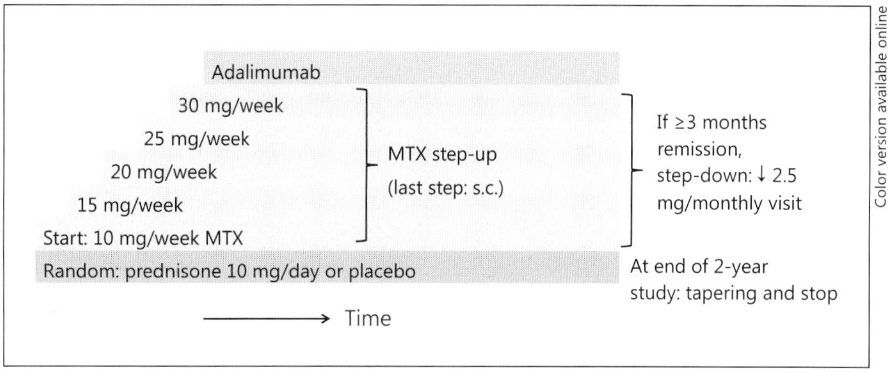

At baseline, year 1 and 2, radiographs of hands and feet were taken and scored by two readers according to the Sharp-van der Heijde score. The primary outcome was radiographic erosive joint damage after 2 years. Secondary outcomes involved clinical improvement.

In CAMERA-II, erosive joint damage after 2 years was limited, but it was significantly less in the strategy group receiving MTX and prednisone (n = 117) compared to the strategy group receiving MTX and placebo (n = 119). The cumulative probability plot of erosion scores at 2 years showed that 78% of all patients in the MTX and prednisone strategy group versus 67% in the MTX and placebo strategy group were still erosion free; of those who did have erosions, erosion scores were higher in the MTX and placebo strategy group (fig. 3), with the exception of the score in 1 patient who already had a high score at baseline.

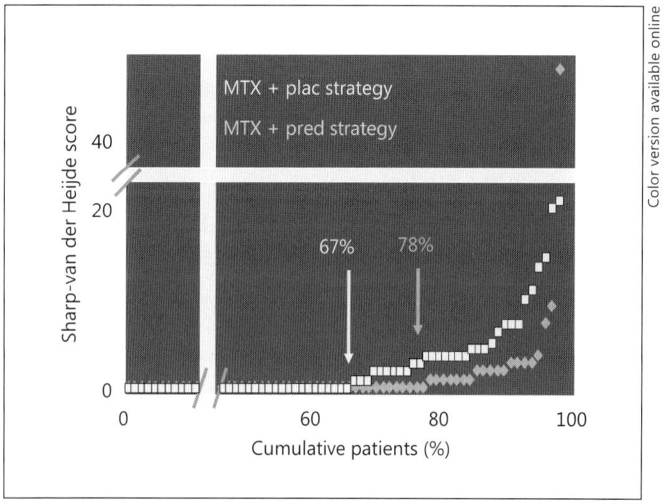

Fig. 3. The cumulative probability plot of erosion scores in CAMERA-II at 2 years. The plot displays the Sharp-van der Heijde scores for erosions (range 0–280) on the y-axis for individual patients, ranked along the x-axis (range 0–100% of patients). Each symbol is 1 patient. Of the patients in the MTX-based strategy with prednisone (MTX + pred strategy), 78% [vs. 67% in the MTX-based strategy with placebo-prednisone (MTX + plac strategy)] were still erosion free at 2 years, and erosion scores of the MTX + plac strategy group were also generally higher. The median erosion score at 2 years was significantly less in the MTX + pred strategy.

The prednisone strategy also yielded more clinical improvement. Occurrence of adverse effects was similar between both strategy groups, with the exception of weight gain, which was less in the placebo strategy group [1.3 (SD 5.3) vs. 2.9 (4.2) kg in the prednisone strategy group] and of nausea and elevated serum alanine and aspartate aminotransferase levels which occurred statistically significantly less in the prednisone strategy group. In an additional analysis, the extra weight gain in the prednisone strategy group seemed largely attributable to a better reduction of disease activity, rather than this being an adverse effect of prednisone [9].

In accordance with study protocol, supplementation with 500 mg of calcium and 400 IU of vitamin D, both usual doses at the time the study was designed, and a bisphosphonate had been given. Dual-energy X-ray absorptiometry of lumbar spine and left hip were performed at baseline, and after 1 and 2 years of treatment. There was no bone loss in either group. Bone mineral density even increased significantly over time in both treatment groups in the lumbar spine with a mean of 2.8% ($p < 0.001$), but not in the hip. Higher age and lower weight at baseline, and higher disease activity scores during the trial, but not glucocorticoid therapy, were associated with a lower bone mineral density at both the lumbar spine and the hip in mixed model analyses [10].

Discussion

Our findings and similar research results from other research groups prove that GCs have disease-modifying properties [11]. This is because they not only suppress signs and symptoms of RA but also slow down the progression of radiological joint damage. The gain of slowing down of radiographic joint damage in patients with early active RA treated with prednisone is not lost after the end of prednisone treatment. In joints with active RA, osteoclasts are directly activated by receptor activator of nuclear factor κB ligand (RANKL) on activated T and B lymphocytes [12]. Downregulation of RANKL within these joints by GCs could be an important mechanism of inhibition of formation of joint erosions. In line with this hypothesis is the finding that in RANKL-knockout mice, experimental arthritis does not cause joint erosions [13], and that denosumab seems to inhibit formation of erosions in RA [14].

The significant difference in radiological scores between the two groups in the Utrecht Study was mainly based on a difference in progression of erosive joint damage (bone) and less on a difference in the decrease in joint space width (cartilage). In several other studies, including CAMERA-II, inhibition of decrease in joint space width was not found [15]. The main difference between the Utrecht Study and these other studies is the more severe (progression of) joint damage in the Utrecht Study, attributable to less tight treatment of RA. This might be an explanation of the discrepancy between these studies regarding joint space width.

Of note, although long-term low-dose GCs seem effective in RA and to be associated with limited radiological progression in observational studies [16], the DMARD effect of GCs has been proven for therapy given during the first 2 years of RA, which is not to say this effect will be absent when treating patients with GCs in a later phase of their disease – this has not yet been investigated.

In the Utrecht Study, vertebral fractures were observed more commonly in the prednisone arm than in the placebo arm (5 vs. 2 patients). Although statistical testing revealed no significant difference, the numbers were small and a type II error cannot be excluded. We feel that the application of GCs, as in the Utrecht Study, which nowadays would be considered unethical, probably leads to bone loss. There was no bone loss in CAMERA-II. We have two explanations for this discrepancy. First, in both arms of the Utrecht Study disease control was not tight, in contrast to in CAMERA-II; inflammatory disease has negative effects on bone, and also on lipids, endothelium, glucose metabolism and infection risk [17–20]. In this way, negative effects of the inflammatory disease are entangled with adverse effects of the GC therapy given for the inflammatory disease. So, in the Utrecht Study, next to the manifold mechanisms of GCs leading to osteoporosis [21], the inflammatory disease not in remission will probably also have contributed to bone loss. Second, in CAMERA-II there was also more adequate use of calcium, vitamin D and bisphosphonates.

Conclusions

In early RA, 10 mg of prednisone daily for 2 years improves the effect of drug therapy and has joint-sparing properties, even if added to a tight control MTX-based strategy aiming for remission. Osteoporosis is rare if inflammation is controlled and patients are given adequate doses of calcium, vitamin D and bisphosphonates, according to national or international guidelines, and if patient compliance for this medication is checked.

References

1 Joint Committee of the Medical Research Council and Nuffield Foundation: A comparison of cortisone and aspirin in the treatment of early cases of rheumatoid arthritis. Br Med J 1954;1:1223–1227.

2 van Everdingen AA, Jacobs JW, Siewertsz van Reesema DR, Bijlsma JW: Low-dose prednisone therapy for patients with early active rheumatoid arthritis: clinical efficacy, disease-modifying properties, and side effects: a randomized, double-blind, placebo-controlled clinical trial. Ann Intern Med 2002; 136:1–12.

3 Bakker MF, Jacobs JW, Welsing PM, et al: Low-dose prednisone inclusion in a methotrexate-based, tight control strategy for early rheumatoid arthritis: a randomized trial. Ann Intern Med 2012;156:329–339.

4 van der Heijde D: How to read radiographs according to the Sharp/van der Heijde method. J Rheumatol 1999;26:743–745.

5 Jacobs JW, van Everdingen AA, Verstappen SM, Bijlsma JW: Follow-up radiographic data on patients with rheumatoid arthritis who participated in a two-year trial of prednisone therapy or placebo. Arthritis Rheum 2006;54:1422–1428.

6 Landewé RB, Boers M, Verhoeven AC, et al: COBRA combination therapy in patients with early rheumatoid arthritis: long-term structural benefits of a brief intervention. Arthritis Rheum 2002;46:347–356.

7 Verstappen SM, Jacobs JW, van der Veen MJ, et al: Intensive treatment with methotrexate in early rheumatoid arthritis: aiming for remission. Computer Assisted Management in Early Rheumatoid Arthritis (CAMERA, an open-label strategy trial). Ann Rheum Dis 2007;66:1443–1449.

8 Bakker MF, Jacobs JW, Welsing PM, et al: Are switches from oral to subcutaneous methotrexate or addition of ciclosporin to methotrexate useful steps in a tight control treatment strategy for rheumatoid arthritis? A post hoc analysis of the CAMERA study. Ann Rheum Dis 2010;69:1849–1852.
9 Jurgens MS, Jacobs JW, Geenen R, et al: Increase of body mass index in a tight controlled methotrexate-based strategy with prednisone in early rheumatoid arthritis: side effect of the prednisone or better control of disease activity? Arthritis Care Res (Hoboken) 2013;65: 88–93.
10 van der Goes MC, Jacobs JW, Jurgens MS, et al: Are changes in bone mineral density different between groups of early rheumatoid arthritis patients treated according to a tight control strategy with or without prednisone if osteoporosis prophylaxis is applied? Osteoporos Int 2013;24:1429–1436.
11 Kirwan J, Power L: Glucocorticoids: action and new therapeutic insights in rheumatoid arthritis. Curr Opin Rheumatol 2007;19:233–237.
12 McQueen F, Naredo E: The 'disconnect' between synovitis and erosion in rheumatoid arthritis: a result of treatment or intrinsic to the disease process itself? Ann Rheum Dis 2011;70:241–244.
13 Gravallese EM, Goldring SR: Cellular mechanisms and the role of cytokines in bone erosions in rheumatoid arthritis. Arthritis Rheum 2000;43:2143–2151.
14 Geusens P: The role of RANK ligand/osteoprotegerin in rheumatoid arthritis. Ther Adv Musculoskelet Dis 2012;4:225–233.
15 Kirwan J, Byron M, Watt I: The relationship between soft tissue swelling, joint space narrowing and erosive damage in hand X-rays of patients with rheumatoid arthritis. Rheumatology (Oxford) 2001;40:297–301.
16 Pincus T, Sokka T, Castrejon I, Cutolo M: Decline of mean initial prednisone dosage from 10.3 to 3.6 mg/day to treat rheumatoid arthritis between 1980 and 2004 in one clinical setting, with long-term effectiveness of dosages less than 5 mg/day. Arthritis Care Res (Hoboken) 2013;65:729–736.
17 Au K, Reed G, Curtis JR, et al: Extended report: high disease activity is associated with an increased risk of infection in patients with rheumatoid arthritis. Ann Rheum Dis 2011; 70:785–791.
18 Wasko MC, Kay J, Hsia EC, Rahman MU: Diabetes mellitus and insulin resistance in patients with rheumatoid arthritis: risk reduction in a chronic inflammatory disease. Arthritis Care Res (Hoboken) 2011;63:512–521.
19 Klarenbeek NB, van der Kooij SM, Huizinga TJ, et al: Blood pressure changes in patients with recent-onset rheumatoid arthritis treated with four different treatment strategies: a post hoc analysis from the BeSt trial. Ann Rheum Dis 2010;69:1342–1345.
20 Peters MJ, Vis M, van Halm VP, et al: Changes in lipid profile during infliximab and corticosteroid treatment in rheumatoid arthritis. Ann Rheum Dis 2007;66:958–961.
21 Bultink IE, Baden M, Lems WF: Glucocorticoid-induced osteoporosis: an update on current pharmacotherapy and future directions. Expert Opin Pharmacother 2013;14:185–197.
22 Jacobs JW: The CAMERA (Computer-Assisted Management in Early Rheumatoid Arthritis) studies. Clin Exp Rheumatol 2012;30:S39–S43.

NeuroImmunoModulation

Neuroimmunomodulation 2015;22:72–82
DOI: 10.1159/000362727

Published online: September 12, 2014

The Safety of Low-Dose Glucocorticoids in Rheumatic Diseases: Results from Observational Studies

Yong Gil Hwang[a] Kenneth Saag[b]

[a]Division of Rheumatology and Clinical Immunology, University of Pittsburgh, Pittsburgh, Pa., and [b]Division of Clinical Immunology and Rheumatology, University of Alabama at Birmingham, Birmingham, Ala., USA

Key Words
Low-dose glucocorticoid · Adverse effect · Rheumatoid arthritis · Safety

Abstract
Glucocorticoids (GC) remain the most commonly used agents for managing inflammatory rheumatic diseases. The adverse effects (AEs) associated with high-dose GCs are well established, but there is a widespread misconception that AEs of high-dose GC therapy (>30 mg of prednisone or equivalent daily) are similar in low-dose therapy (≤7.5 mg of prednisone equivalent a day). Although high-quality evidence on AEs of low-dose GC therapy is still incomplete, risks and safety of low-dose GC therapy in rheumatic diseases are reviewed based on current evidence by category, including musculoskeletal, cardiovascular, infectious, gastrointestinal, neuropsychiatric, endocrine and metabolic, dermatologic, and ophthalmologic AEs. Recommendations concerning monitoring AEs with low-dose GC therapy are provided for each category of AEs on the basis of our literature review and clinical experience. There is emerging evidence that low-dose GCs are associated with a much lower level of AEs, which would allow their use over long periods in patients with rheumatic disease who gain clinical effectiveness and well-being from their use. Nonetheless, knowledge and understanding of AEs from low-dose GCs is vital to maximize benefits and minimize risks to patients.

Introduction

Since the introduction of glucocorticoids (GCs) in the 1950s, they have been widely used in a large variety of inflammatory diseases. Adverse effects (AEs) of high-dose GCs are well established and have limited their use, but these AEs are much less common with low-dose GCs. In this review, we will focus on low-dose use of GC treatment, defined as a treatment with ≤7.5 mg of prednisone equivalent a day from observational studies, although a dose <5 mg of prednisone per day may also be recognized as a low dose. Of note, GCs in the low-dose range occupy less than 50% of the GC receptors and are less associated with non-genomic effects [1]. In this review, we define a medium dose as >7.5–30 mg/day and high-dose GC therapy as >30 mg of prednisone or equivalent daily.

Although high-quality evidence on AEs of low-dose GC therapy is often scarce and at times conflicting, we

KARGER

E-Mail karger@karger.com
www.karger.com/nim

1021–7401/14/0222–0072$39.50/0

Kenneth Saag
820 Faculty Office Tower
510 20th Street South
Birmingham, AL 35294 (USA)
E-Mail kenneth.saag@ccc.uab.edu

present the risks and safety of low-dose GC therapy in rheumatic diseases based on the best current knowledge available from observational studies. Since the vast majority of available data on GCs are retrospective, efforts have been made recently to define the AEs of chronic GC treatment in lower dosages based on prospective cohort studies [2, 3]. Although the EULAR Task Force on GCs formulated recommendations for the monitoring of low-dose GC-related AEs, it is difficult to systematically assess some AEs, such as psychological or behavioral AEs. All observational data on this topic include persistent problems with confounding [4]. Furthermore, it is often difficult to differentiate AEs of low-dose GC therapy from those occurring from the underlying GC-requiring diseases or other co-morbidities. Specifically, physicians are more inclined to treat patients with more active and severe diseases with GCs, an example of confounding by indication [5]. Randomized controlled clinical trials (RCTs) eliminate this source of confounding but bring with them the absence of real-world effectiveness, small sample sizes, limited duration of follow-up, and often a lack of systematic evaluation of certain AEs. Data from RCTs will not be covered in this review but are discussed in the article by Santiago and Da Silva in this special issue.

General Determinants of GC AEs

The occurrence of AEs is heavily dependent on the dose and duration of GC therapy. Other factors that may influence both the therapeutic benefit and AEs include the patient's age, timing of doses during the day, individual differences in GC metabolism, and rate of GC clearance. A pharmacokinetic alteration seen in the elderly may contribute to the increased incidence of AEs from chronic GC therapy in older adults [6, 7]. It is believed that giving GCs as a single dose early in the morning, or in an alternate-day regimen, leads to less Cushing's syndrome or pituitary suppression [8]. However, alternate-day therapy is usually unsuccessful in controlling underlying diseases, such as rheumatoid arthritis (RA).

A threshold dose or duration has not been well described for most AEs of GCs. There appear to be two distinct dose-related patterns of AEs based on self-reported health problems evaluated in 1,066 RA patients by Huscher et al. [9]. A 'linear' increase with increasing dose was found for a Cushingoid phenotype, ecchymosis, leg edema, mycosis, parchment-like skin, shortness of breath and sleep disturbance. A 'threshold pattern' describing an elevated frequency of events beyond a certain threshold

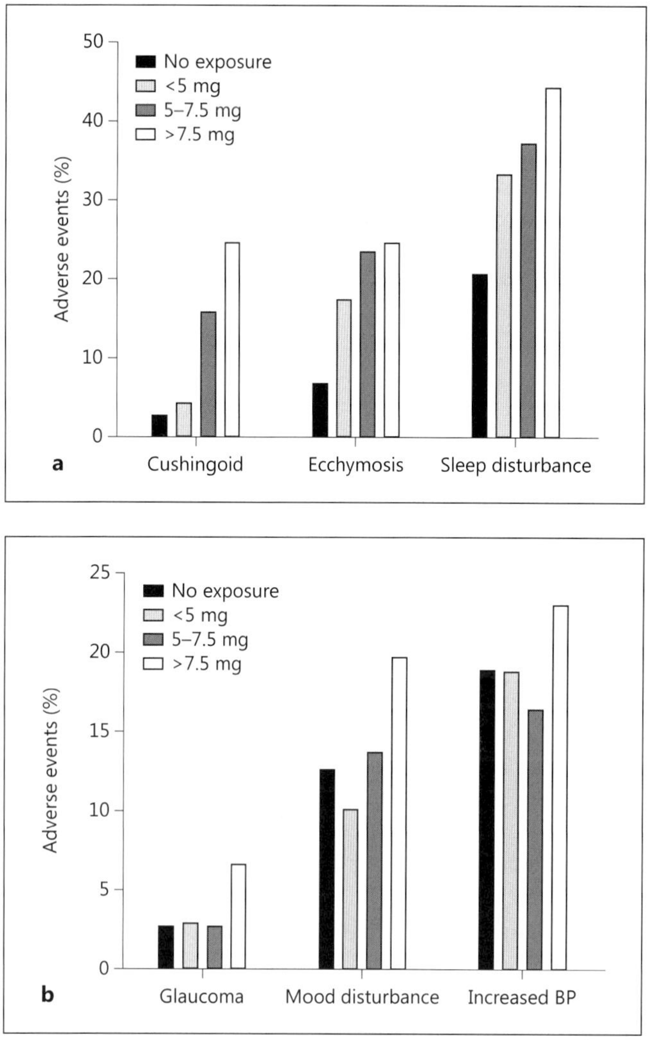

Fig. 1. Two distinct dose-related patterns, linear (**a**) and threshold (**b**), of adverse events were observed from self-reported health problems relating to dose and duration of GC intake in unselected patients with RA from routine practice (n = 1,066) [adapted from 9].

value was observed at medium-to-high dose for glaucoma, depression/listlessness and increases in blood pressure (BP). Dosages of 5 mg/day or more were associated with epistaxis and weight gain. A very-low-dose GC threshold was seen for cataract (<5 mg/day; fig. 1).

The underlying GC-requiring disease and co-morbidities are important factors independently associated with GC AEs. While even low-dose GC therapy likely increases osteoporosis risk, underlying diseases such as RA or systemic lupus erythematosus (SLE) also increase the risk of osteoporosis. Co-morbidities, such as COPD and diabetes, could increase risk of serious infection and altered glucose metabolism, and could lead to polypharmacy with risk for GC drug interactions. Although significant interactions between GCs and other medications have been well documented, there are no adequate prospective studies of these interactions. Patients and rheumatologists share concordant worries about mangy AEs, such as osteoporosis, diabetes and cardiovascular (CV) diseases. However, frequent but less serious AEs (e.g. skin thinning, Cushingoid appearance) may be of greater concern to patients than to physicians [10].

Musculoskeletal AEs

Osteoporosis

GC therapy is the most common cause of secondary osteoporosis. Higher dose and longer duration of GC use are strongly associated with the risk of fractures [11, 12]. However, no consensus exists regarding a safe average or cumulative GC dosage with regard to bone, as wide individual variation is seen. The effects of long-term high-dose GCs on bone mineral density (BMD) are clear, but the effects of lower-dose GCs in patients with rheumatic diseases remain somewhat controversial.

In a meta-analysis in 2008, low-dose GC use resulted in a moderate worsening in lumbar BMD compared with controls, whereas femoral BMD was not significantly decreased. Subgroup analysis of BMD data performed on a change-from-baseline basis showed that GCs had a clear effect on both lumbar and femoral BMDs [13]. However, there are few data on the reversibility of this risk after cessation of GC therapy. In a retrospective cohort study in a general medical practice setting in the UK (using data from the General Practice Research Database, GPRD), a dose dependence of fracture risk was observed. With a standardized daily dose of <2.5 mg of prednisolone, hip fracture relative risk (RR) was 0.99 (95% CI 0.82–1.20) relative to controls, rising to 1.77 (1.55–2.02) at daily doses of 2.5–7.5 mg, and 2.27 (1.94–2.66) at doses of 7.5 mg or greater. For vertebral fracture, the RRs were 1.55 (1.20–2.01), 2.59 (2.16–3.10) and 5.18 (4.25–6.31), respectively. All fracture risks declined toward baseline rapidly after cessation of oral GC treatment [14].

In a recent study of the effect of GC dose on FRAX®-derived fracture probabilities in a UK setting (using data from GPRD), a new rule was formulated. For very-low-dose exposure (<2.5 mg daily of prednisolone or equivalent), the probability of a major fracture decreased by about 20% depending on age, but for doses between 2.5 and 7.5 mg daily, the unadjusted FRAX value can be used [15]. In summary, although osteoporosis may be aggravated by low-dose GC therapy, very-low-dose exposure appears not to be associated with increased risk of osteoporosis from our clinical experience.

Osteonecrosis

Although numerous reports describe osteonecrosis after high-dose GC therapy, it is difficult to determine the relative contributions of the GC treatment and the underlying disease [16]. To our knowledge, there is no evidence on the occurrence of osteonecrosis during low-dose GC therapy. Nonetheless, it is generally accepted that in patients treated with low doses of GC, osteonecrosis is very uncommon.

Myopathy

Comparison of muscle biopsies from 22 RA patients who had been on long-term low-dose GC therapy with 15 patients who never received GCs showed a low proportion of type I fiber, and reduced type I and type II mean fiber areas [17]. In a separate study by the same investigative group, compared to patients with RA who had never been treated with GCs, the reduction in knee extensor strength was 37 and 28%, respectively ($p < 0.001$ and $p < 0.01$). The mean walking speed in patients with GC treatment was 0.9 m/s, a 36% reduction compared with patients who had not received GCs ($p < 0.01$) [18].

The clinical picture of GC-associated myopathy can be very difficult to distinguish from the effects of the underlying disease, especially in the case of musculoskeletal conditions. To our knowledge, there are no reports of myopathy in controlled studies with GC therapy <10 mg/day of prednisone equivalent, and it is believed that myopathy is exceedingly rare with low-dose GC therapy [19–23]. It should be noted that GC therapy may trigger attacks of normokalemic or hypokalemic periodic paralysis. This is very rare, but GCs should be administered with caution in patients with periodic paralysis [24].

Cardiovascular AEs

Dyslipidemia, Atherosclerosis and Ischemic Heart Disease

GC treatment, especially high cumulative GC exposure, is regarded as a risk factor for increasing unfavorable lipid profiles and accelerated coronary atherosclerosis [25]. In rheumatic diseases, lipid metabolism may be altered by systemic inflammation, environmental lifestyle factors, drug therapy and several genetic factors. Several studies in SLE patients reported an association between treatment with high doses of GCs and development of an atherogenic plasma lipid profile, but these findings may be confounded by indication and the underlying disease [26–28]. By contrast, low-dose GC therapy in RA patients is generally associated with an increase in HDL, without increasing LDL or triglyceride – changes which may be favorable [29–31].

In a cross-sectional study of 398 patients with RA [32], metabolic syndrome was found in 40.1% of patients; the prevalence in patients with no GC exposure was 37.9%, versus 40.7% with long-term low-dose exposure, versus 50% with long-term medium-dose exposure (p = 0.241). The odds ratio (OR) for metabolic syndrome comparing medium with low dose (OR = 1.64; 95% CI 0.92–2.92) [32] was higher, though not statistically significant. In a recent systematic literature review [33], low-dose GC in RA patients showed a protective effect on serum lipid profile but no effect on atherosclerosis.

Increased CV events are observed in rheumatic patients who were exposed to higher cumulative exposure and higher average daily dosage of GC [34, 35]. In the above systemic review of low-dose GC therapy [33], somewhat in contrast with the lipid findings, four out of six studies reviewed found that low-dose GC therapy was associated with major CV events, including myocardial infarction (HR = 1.7; 95% CI 1.2–2.3), stroke (OR = 4.36; 95% CI 1.60–11.90, for GC between 6 and 10 mg/day), mortality (HR = 2.03; 95% CI 1.25–3.32) and a composite index of CV events (in the group of rheumatoid factor-positive RA, HR = 2.21; 95% CI 1.22–4.00). However, two studies did not find any significant association between low-dose GC exposure and mortality (OR = 2.25; 95% CI 0.29–102.5) or a composite index of CV events (OR = 1.3; 95% CI 0.8–2.0). Although the literature reviewed did not show statistically significant associations between low-dose GC exposure and CV risk factors, a trend of increasing major CV events was identified [33]. A recent incident RA cohort in British Columbia, Canada, found that myocardial infarction risk increased by 13% for each 5 mg/day increase in dose, and by 10% per additional year on GCs [36]. In contrast, the use of low-dose GCs did not increase the CV risk in a large population-based study from Scotland [37]. Thus, the effects of low-dose GC on atherosclerosis and progression of CV disease remain incompletely characterized.

Water and Electrolyte Balance, Edema, Heart Failure and Hypertension

GCs at high doses can cause hypernatremia, hypokalemia, a marked anti-natriuresis and expansion of extracellular fluid and plasma volume. They raise BP in humans and animals through mineralocorticoid effects [38]. However, synthetic GCs (prednisone, prednisolone and dexamethasone) have little mineralocorticoid effect and induce kaliuresis and natriuresis without any change in plasma volume [39, 40]. Data on the occurrence of edema during low-dose GC treatment is scarce, although there was a linearly rising frequency of leg edema with increasing dose in self-reported health problems (no GC in the past 12 months, <5, 5–7.5 and >7.5 mg/day: 9.5, 11.6, 20.2 and 26.2%, respectively) [9, 41, 42].

Follow-up of 195 patients undergoing low-dose GC therapy did not show any relationship between change of BP and either dose of corticosteroid or duration of therapy [43]. RCTs also did not reveal an increased risk of hypertension in patients treated with low-dose GCs [41, 44–48]. It is important to note that the studies we identified did not document use of special measurements evaluating BP, edema or electrolyte disorders with low-dose GC therapy. Thus, there remains some uncertainty about the association of low-dose GCs with changes in BP and water balance.

Infectious AEs

GC therapy is strongly associated with an increased risk of serious infections in patients with rheumatic diseases, with increased risk associated with increased doses [49]. However, disease severity is an important confounding factor for the GC-associated infectious complications observed in clinical practice. In a total of 7,971 patients with RA enrolled in the Consortium of Rheumatology Researchers of North America (CORRONA) registry who were prescribed methotrexate, TNF antagonists or other disease-modifying anti-rheumatic drugs, low-dose prednisone use overall was not associated with risk of infection [50]. However, low-dose prednisone and TNF antagonists (but not methotrexate) increased the risk of opportunistic infections. An analysis of combined administrative databases, including Medicare, identified over 1,100 infections among a population of over 16,000 individuals with immune-mediated diseases. For GC doses in the 0–5 mg per day range, the adjusted HR was 1.32 (95% CI 1.1–1.58) for serious bacterial infections [51].

In a meta-analysis of 71 controlled clinical trials involving over 2,000 patients randomly allocated to systemic GCs in the setting of different diseases, an RR for the overall infectious complications was 1.6 (95% CI 1.3–1.9). The rate was not increased in patients given a daily dose of <10 mg or a cumulative dose of <700 mg of prednisone [52]. By contrast, a recent systematic review identified 15 studies assessing the infection risk of low-dose GC therapy in RA patients and did not find consistent associations between infection risk and low-dose GC treatment [53]. In a double-blind RCT conducted over 12 weeks in 143 patients with active RA comparing 3 mg of budesonide daily, 9 mg of budesonide daily, 7.5 mg of prednisolone daily and placebo, Kirwan et al. [46] reported that respiratory infection and viral infections were more frequently observed in the GC group (respiratory infections in 17/112 in the GC group vs. 1/31 in the placebo group; viral infection in 5/112 in the GC group vs. 0/31 in the placebo group). However, an RCT of 242 patients with early active RA comparing 7.5 mg/day of prednisolone or no prednisolone for 2 years reported no significant difference in pneumonitis and fever between the two groups [54]. In a nested case-control analysis based on a cohort of 16,207 patients with RA aged over 65 years from administrative data, GC therapy was associated with an adjusted RR of 1.20 (95% CI 1.15–1.25) for non-serious infection. A dose response was seen as the adjusted RR increased from 1.10 (<5 mg/day) to 1.85 for doses greater than 20 mg/day. While the RR is low at 1.20, the absolute risk was high, with one additional infection seen for every 13 patients treated with GCs for 1 year [55]. In summary, the literature suggests the risk for infections could be increased in low-dose GC users.

Gastrointestinal AEs

Peptic Ulcer Disease

The relationship between non-steroidal anti-inflammatory drugs (NSAIDs) and peptic ulcer disease is well established. However, the literature on GCs is more limited than that on NSAIDs, and the association between GC use and risk of peptic ulcer disease has been controversial [56, 57]. In a nested case-control study that included 1,415 patients who were admitted for gastric or duodenal ulcer or for upper gastrointestinal hemorrhage of unknown cause, and 7,063 control subjects randomly selected from Medicaid, the estimated RR for the development of peptic ulcer disease among current users of oral corticosteroids was 2.0 (95% CI 1.3–3.0). However, those concurrently receiving GCs and NSAIDs had a risk for peptic ulcer disease that was 15 times greater than that of non-users of either drug (concurrent NSAID user estimated RR 4.4; 95% CI 2.0–9.7; NSAID nonusers RR 1.1; 95% CI 0.5–2.1) [58].

In a nested case-control analysis using data from GPRD in the UK [59], the overall adjusted OR for upper gastrointestinal complications associated with current use of oral GCs alone was 1.8 (95% CI 1.3–2.4) compared with non-users. Concurrent use of GCs with low-medium and high NSAID doses, respectively, produced ORs of 4.0 (95% CI 1.3–12.0) and 12.7 (95% CI 6.2–26.1), compared with non-users [59]. A more recent case-control study based on the Health Improvement Network UK primary care database showed that, compared with low-dose aspirin monotherapy, the risk of upper gastrointestinal bleeding was significantly increased when low-dose aspirin was co-administered with high-dose oral GCs (RR 4.43; 95% CI 2.10–9.34); this was not apparent with low-dose oral GCs (RR 1.01; 95% CI 0.58–1.77) [60]. In summary, peptic ulcer disease is a very rare complication of low-dose GC therapy without concomitant use of NSAIDs, and it should not be considered an absolute contraindication when GC therapy is indicated [61].

Pancreatitis

Although high-dose GC therapy is implicated as one of many potential causes of pancreatitis, evidence for such an association is somewhat weak. In a case series of 8 patients over a 10-year period with pancreatitis and SLE, all 8 patients received therapeutic doses of GCs as part of their treatment for SLE and pancreatitis. All patients manifested both clinical and biochemical resolution of their pancreatitis with the administration of GCs [62]. A nationwide population-based case control study in Sweden found over 6,000 episodes of pancreatitis. The risk of acute pancreatitis was increased among current users of oral GCs compared with non-users (OR 1.53; 95% CI 1.27–1.84) with the risk highest in the first 2 weeks after drug administration. Regrettably, the Swedish drug registry used does not provide information about drug dose, thus it is not possible to discern whether this association was dose dependent [63]. In summary, the risk of developing pancreatitis is probably very low and not independently associated with low-dose GC therapy.

Neuropsychiatric AEs

High-dose GC therapy has been associated with a variety of neuropsychiatric side effects, such as insomnia, depression, hypomania or euphoria, confusion and memory problems. There is substantial variability in the reported incidence of neuropsychiatric AEs largely because of unpredictable reactions, the wide range of GC doses, diverse patient groups, and differences in the methodology of assessing these AEs. In a meta-analysis of 11 uncontrolled studies involving 935 adult patients, severe psychiatric reactions were reported in approximately 5% of steroid-treated patients, and mild-to-moderate reactions occurred in about 28% [64]. The Boston Collaborative Drug Surveillance Program monitored 718 prednisone-treated patients and recorded a 1.3% (6/463) incidence of psychiatric disturbance at 40 mg/day or less, 4.6% at 41–80 mg/day, and 18.4% with more than 80 mg/day [65].

Although disturbances of mood, cognition, sleep and behavior, as well as frank delirium or even psychosis are possible, the most common AEs of short-term GC therapy are euphoria and hypomania. By contrast, long-term therapy tends to be associated with depressive symptoms [66]. In a case-control study of 20 patients receiving long-term low-dose GC (7.5 mg/day of prednisone for >6 months) and 14 control subjects, 12 (60%) of 20 GC-treated patients met diagnostic criteria for a lifetime prednisone-induced mood disorder [67]. In a self-report of health problems relating to dose and duration of GC intake of 1,066 patients with RA, sleep disturbance increased linearly with increasing dose and depression/emotional lability were reported more frequently at doses greater than 7.5 mg/day (fig. 1) [9].

In a prospective cohort of 92 patients with SLE, factors predictive of psychosis were low serum levels of albumin, complement and creatinine, history of anxiety disorders, and a family history of psychiatric illnesses. However, after multivariate adjustment, only hypoalbuminemia remained significant [68].

In self-reported health problems relating to the dose and duration of GC intake of 1,066 patients with RA, Huscher et al. [9] recently showed that sleep disturbance increases linearly with increasing dose and depression/emotional lability were reported more frequently at doses of over 7.5 mg/day (fig. 1). In the double-blind RCT by Kirwan et al. [46] described above, depression and mood swings were more frequently reported in the GC group (depression in 20/112 in the GC group vs. 4/31 in the placebo group; mood swings in 16/112 in the GC group vs. 6/31 in the placebo group). However, the exact incidence of such symptoms in rheumatic patients who received low-dose GC therapy cannot be determined from clinical trials. The literature on the prevention and treatment of potential GC-induced adverse psychiatric effects is poorly developed [69]. In summary, GC-induced psychiatric AEs are unpredictable in individual patients, although dosage appears to be related to the incidence of AEs but not to the timing, severity or duration of these effects.

Endocrine and Metabolic AEs

Diabetes and Glucose Intolerance

Medium- to high-dose GC therapy is well established to cause impaired glucose tolerance and insulin resistance. In a case-control study of 128 SLE patients who were categorized as either prednisone non-users (n = 41), low-dose (n = 71) or medium-dose (n = 16) users, daily medium-dose GC use but not low-dose use increased insulin levels and insulin resistance [70]. In a population-based case control study, the OR for development of hyperglycemia requiring treatment in patients using 0.25–2.5 mg of prednisone equivalent a day was 1.77, and the magnitude of risk increased substantially with increasing GC dose [71].

Development of new-onset diabetes after starting low-dose GC treatment is rare, but progression of preceding glucose intolerance to diabetes is more possible [4]. In a long-term observational study in patients with RA (n = 290), less than 3% of patients developed diabetes while receiving low-dose prednisone (prednisone <5 mg/day) [5]. To our knowledge, no studies are available on the specific effects of low-dose GC in diabetic patients.

Weight Gain and Fat Redistribution

The incidence of iatrogenic Cushingoid syndrome is dose dependent and, in general, does not become evident until after at least 1 month of GC therapy [72]. The development of Cushingoid features (fat redistribution, buffalo hump and moon face) and weight gain are particularly displeasing to patients [73]. Therapeutic doses of GC induce obesity primarily by increasing energy intake, an effect which may be related to the capacity of GCs to act directly or indirectly on the central regulation of appetite [74]. In the observational study by Huscher et al. [9] described above, a dose of 5 mg/day or greater was associated with weight gain, and the frequency of Cushingoid features was linearly associated with increasing dose (fig. 1).

In a population-based assessment of 2,466 long-term GC users, all AEs demonstrated a strong dose-dependent association with cumulative GC use. Among users of low-dose therapy (n = 670), increasing duration of use was significantly associated with weight gain (90-day increase in duration of use; OR = 1.09, 95% CI 1.01–1.18) [73]. In RCTs with low-dose GC, increase in body weight and development of Cushingoid features are described, but the data are conflicting [41, 44–46, 48]. Although diminished Cushingoid side effects with alternate-day treatment were observed in liver transplant recipients [75], the only established preventive measures are shorter and lower doses of GC.

Interference with Hypothalamic-Pituitary-Adrenal Axis Hormone Secretion

GCs in high doses suppress the hypothalamic-pituitary-adrenal (HPA) axis, alter hypothalamic gonadotropin-releasing hormone (GnRH) secretion, and decrease basal and GnRH-stimulated luteinizing hormone secretion from the pituitary, leading to decreased estrogen and testosterone. Observational studies indicate that therapy with low-dose GCs does not result in residual pituitary-adrenal hypofunction, and patients receiving <5 mg of prednisone daily have normal HPA axis response [76–79]. In the study of double-blind RCT conducted by Kirwan et al. [80], as described above, low doses of a GC resulted in depression of baseline and ACTH-stimulated cortisol levels after 12 weeks of therapy, although the responsiveness of the HPA axis in individual patients generally remained within the normal range. If withdrawal of GCs is indicated, gradual reduction in dose is appropriate for these patients, especially those who have a Cushingoid appearance.

The effect of chronic GC therapy on serum testosterone and estrogen level predominates in old men and reductions in circulating estradiol concentrations could be implicated in the pathogenesis of GC-induced osteoporosis in men [81, 82]. However, data from clinical trials with low-dose GC are scarce, and this question has not been systematically studied.

Dermatologic AEs

Most of the cutaneous AEs – including skin atrophy, acne, purpura, easy bruisability and impaired wound healing – are not considered serious by the physician, but they are among the most common AEs reported by the patient [2, 9]. Catabolic effects on the skin, including skin atrophy and formation of telangiectasia, mainly result from the effect of GCs on keratinocytes and fibroblasts. GC-associated purpura is often observed in the sun-exposed areas of the dorsum of the hand and forearm. It is believed that decreased vascular structural integrity is probably a key determinant of purpura and easy bruisability in GC-treated patients [83].

In a self-reported health survey assessing the dose and duration of GC intake of 1,066 patients with RA [9], an increased frequency of bruising was reported even in patients taking less than 5 mg/day of GCs over a course of over 6 months (17.4%) compared with the group with no GC exposure in the previous 12 months (6.8%). Bruising was increased with higher dosage (fig. 1) [9]. Delayed wound healing seems uncommon at a low dose, but there are no strong data on prevalence. RCTs with low-dose GC therapy have not reported on the occurrence of skin atrophy. To our knowledge, there is little or no evidence supporting an increased occurrence of acne, hirsutism or alopecia during low-dose GC therapy [41, 44, 46, 54]. Skin thinning and bruising appear the only common AEs during low-dose GC therapy, but most patients find these AEs a tolerable 'trade-off' for a greater sense of well-being.

Ophthalmologic AEs

Cataract

GC-induced cataracts usually occur in a posterior subcapsular location, often bilaterally. They characteristically involve aberrant migrating lens epithelial cells and a central posterior location [84]. Cataracts often occur after prolonged GC use, but disagreement exists concerning the effects of total dose, intensity of dose and duration of administration on cataract formation.

In an observational study of 112 RA patients on low-dose (6.1 ± 3.1 mg/day) long-term (6.2 ± 4.6 years) prednisone, 15% were found to have cataracts, compared with 4.5% of 112 matched RA patients not using prednisone [85]. However, an increased risk for cataract was not reported in RCTs with low-dose GC therapy, and most studies are dependent on self-reported data [41, 44]. There is no evidence that alternate-day treatment reduces the risk and it is believed that cataract formation is irreversible.

Glaucoma and Increased Intraocular Pressure

It is well known that GCs increase the risk of glaucoma by raising the intraocular pressure when administered exogenously, and in certain conditions of increased endogenous production (e.g. Cushing's syndrome). The incidence of increased intraocular pressure with GC tends to increase in individuals with pre-existing glaucoma, age over 40 years, or certain systemic diseases (e.g. diabetes mellitus, high myopia), as well as among relatives of patients with primary open angle glaucoma [86]. In an observational study of 3,792 RA patients enrolled in the German National Database (NDB) [9], glaucoma was found in 3.4% of RA patients who were not exposed to GCs in the past 12 months ver-

Table 1. GC adverse event-monitoring recommendations

Adverse event	Monitoring recommendations
Musculoskeletal	
Osteoporosis	Follow national guidelines [87] but consider the underlying disease as a key co-factor in osteoporosis development.
Osteonecrosis and myopathy	No specific monitoring recommended.
CV	
Dyslipidemia, atherosclerosis	Standard assessment of CV risk factors required.
Electrolyte disturbances	
Hypertension	
Infectious	Standard care with heightened vigilance for infectious sequelae and encourage patients to seek prompt medical care for febrile illnesses.
Gastrointestinal	
Peptic ulcer disease	Avoid concomitant use of NSAIDs.
Pancreatitis	No specific monitoring recommended.
Neuropsychiatric	No specific monitoring recommended.
Endocrine and metabolic	
Diabetes and glucose intolerance	No specific monitoring recommended.
Weight gain and fat redistribution	Gradual dose reduction for patients with a Cushingoid appearance.
Interference with hormone secretion	No specific monitoring recommended.
Dermatologic	No specific monitoring recommended.
Ophthalmologic	
Cataract	No specific monitoring recommended.
Glaucoma	Identify other risk factors and educate patients.

sus 4.6% of RA patients who were exposed to GC >7.5 mg/day for more than 6 months. In the same database, the frequency of self-reported glaucoma from 1,066 RA patients increased only at a dosage >7.5 mg/day [9]. Data from clinical trials are conflicting and endpoints are not adequately defined, although ophthalmologic examination in a 2-year follow-up showed increased incidence of glaucoma (n = 166, 3 in the GC group, 0 in the placebo group) [41, 44].

Conclusion

Although there is growing evidence from prospective studies, the frequency of many AEs associated with low-dose GC use remains elusive. Overall, concerns of low-dose GC toxicity are prevalent among physicians, but these may be overestimated based on the existing guidelines and what is currently known. Given the fact that GCs have disease-modifying potential, clear guidelines about the toxicity of low-dose GC may prove helpful. The EULAR Task Force on GCs formulated recommendations for the monitoring of low-dose GC-related AEs, based on reports of GC-related AEs. However, despite the endemic use of low-dose GC therapy in rheumatic diseases, evidence on the toxicity of low-dose GC is surprisingly weak and data from appropriately designed clinical trials is still lacking for most AE outcomes. From our literature review and clinical experience, table 1 provides brief summary of our recommendations on monitoring AEs with low-dose GC therapy. As is true in nearly all areas of medicine, care for individuals using GCs in the rheumatic diseases should be based on shared decisions between a patient and a physician to maximize benefit and minimize individual risk.

References

1 Buttgereit F, da Silva JA, Boers M, Burmester GR, Cutolo M, Jacobs J, Kirwan J, Kohler L, Van Riel P, Vischer T, Bijlsma JW: Standardised nomenclature for glucocorticoid dosages and glucocorticoid treatment regimens: current questions and tentative answers in rheumatology. Ann Rheum Dis 2002; 61:718–722.

2 Da Silva JA, Jacobs JW, Kirwan JR, Boers M, Saag KG, Ines LB, de Koning EJ, Buttgereit F, Cutolo M, Capell H, Rau R, Bijlsma JW: Safety of low-dose glucocorticoid treatment in rheumatoid arthritis: published evidence and prospective trial data. Ann Rheum Dis 2006; 65:285–293.

3 Hoes JN, Jacobs JW, Boers M, Boumpas D, Buttgereit F, Caeyers N, Choy EH, Cutolo M, Da Silva JA, Esselens G, Guillevin L, Hafstrom I, Kirwan JR, Rovensky J, Russell A, Saag KG, Svensson B, Westhovens R, Zeidler H, Bijlsma JW: Eular evidence-based recommendations on the management of systemic glucocorticoid therapy in rheumatic diseases. Ann Rheum Dis 2007;66:1560–1567.

4 van der Goes MC, Jacobs JW, Boers M, Andrews T, Blom-Bakkers MA, Buttgereit F, Caeyers N, Cutolo M, Da Silva JA, Guillevin L, Kirwan JR, Rovensky J, Severijns G, Webber S, Westhovens R, Bijlsma JW: Monitoring adverse events of low-dose glucocorticoid therapy: EULAR recommendations for clinical trials and daily practice. Ann Rheum Dis 2010;69:1913–1919.

5 Pincus T, Sokka T, Castrejon I, Cutolo M: Decline of mean initial prednisone dosage from 10.3 to 3.6 mg/day to treat rheumatoid arthritis between 1980 and 2004 in one clinical setting, with long-term effectiveness of dosages less than 5 mg/day. Arthritis Care Res (Hoboken) 2013;65:729–736.

6 Fisher DA: Adverse effects of topical corticosteroid use. West J Med 1995;162:123–126.

7 Tornatore KM, Logue G, Venuto RC, Davis PJ: Pharmacokinetics of methylprednisolone in elderly and young healthy males. J Am Geriatr Soc 1994;42:1118–1122.

8 Cutolo M: Hormone therapy in rheumatic diseases. Curr Opin Rheumatol 2010;22:257–263.

9 Huscher D, Thiele K, Gromnica-Ihle E, Hein G, Demary W, Dreher R, Zink A, Buttgereit F: Dose-related patterns of glucocorticoid-induced side effects. Ann Rheum Dis 2009;68: 1119–1124.

10 van der Goes MC, Jacobs JW, Boers M, Andrews T, Blom-Bakkers MA, Buttgereit F, Caeyers N, Choy EH, Cutolo M, Da Silva JA, Guillevin L, Holland M, Kirwan JR, Rovensky J, Saag KG, Severijns G, Webber S, Westhovens R, Bijlsma JW: Patient and rheumatologist perspectives on glucocorticoids: an exercise to improve the implementation of the European League Against Rheumatism (EULAR) recommendations on the management of systemic glucocorticoid therapy in rheumatic diseases. Ann Rheum Dis 2010;69:1015–1021.

11 Van Staa TP, Laan RF, Barton IP, Cohen S, Reid DM, Cooper C: Bone density threshold and other predictors of vertebral fracture in patients receiving oral glucocorticoid therapy. Arthritis Rheum 2003;48:3224–3229.

12 Steinbuch M, Youket TE, Cohen S: Oral glucocorticoid use is associated with an increased risk of fracture. Osteoporos Int 2004;15:323–328.

13 Lee YH, Woo JH, Choi SJ, Ji JD, Song GG: Effects of low-dose corticosteroids on the bone mineral density of patients with rheumatoid arthritis: a meta-analysis. J Investig Med 2008; 56:1011–1018.

14 Van Staa TP, Leufkens HG, Abenhaim L, Zhang B, Cooper C: Use of oral corticosteroids and risk of fractures. J Bone Miner Res 2000;15:993–1000.

15 Kanis JA, Johansson H, Oden A, McCloskey EV: Guidance for the adjustment of FRAX according to the dose of glucocorticoids. Osteoporos Int 2011;22:809–816.

16 Gebhard KL, Maibach HI: Relationship between systemic corticosteroids and osteonecrosis. Am J Clin Dermatol 2001;2:377–388.

17 Danneskiold-Samsoe B, Grimby G: The influence of prednisone on the muscle morphology and muscle enzymes in patients with rheumatoid arthritis. Clin Sci (Lond) 1986;71: 693–701.

18 Danneskiold-Samsoe B, Grimby G: The relationship between the leg muscle strength and physical capacity in patients with rheumatoid arthritis, with reference to the influence of corticosteroids. Clin Rheumatol 1986;5:468–474.

19 Hollingworth P, de Vere Tyndall A, Ansell BM, Platts-Mills T, Gumpel JM, Mertin J, Smith DS, Denman AM: Intensive immunosuppression versus prednisolone in the treatment of connective tissue diseases. Ann Rheum Dis 1982;41:557–562.

20 Jover JA, Hernandez-Garcia C, Morado IC, Vargas E, Banares A, Fernandez-Gutierrez B: Combined treatment of giant-cell arteritis with methotrexate and prednisone: a randomized, double-blind, placebo-controlled trial. Ann Intern Med 2001;134:106–114.

21 Spiera RF, Mitnick HJ, Kupersmith M, Richmond M, Spiera H, Peterson MG, Paget SA: A prospective, double-blind, randomized, placebo controlled trial of methotrexate in the treatment of giant cell arteritis (GCA). Clin Exp Rheumatol 2001;19:495–501.

22 Hunder GG, Sheps SG, Allen GL, Joyce JW: Daily and alternate-day corticosteroid regimens in treatment of giant cell arteritis: comparison in a prospective study. Ann Intern Med 1975;82:613–618.

23 Mazlumzadeh M, Hunder GG, Easley KA, Calamia KT, Matteson EL, Griffing WL, Younge BR, Weyand CM, Goronzy JJ: Treatment of giant cell arteritis using induction therapy with high-dose glucocorticoids: a double-blind, placebo-controlled, randomized prospective clinical trial. Arthritis Rheum 2006;54:3310–3318.

24 Arzel-Hezode M, McGoey S, Sternberg D, Vicart S, Eymard B, Fontaine B: Glucocorticoids may trigger attacks in several types of periodic paralysis. Neuromuscul Disord 2009;19:217–219.

25 Becker DM, Chamberlain B, Swank R, Hegewald MG, Girardet R, Baughman KL, Kwiterovich PO, Pearson TA, Ettinger WH, Renlund D: Relationship between corticosteroid exposure and plasma lipid levels in heart transplant recipients. Am J Med 1988;85:632–638.

26 MacGregor AJ, Dhillon VB, Binder A, Forte CA, Knight BC, Betteridge DJ, Isenberg DA: Fasting lipids and anticardiolipin antibodies as risk factors for vascular disease in systemic lupus erythematosus. Ann Rheum Dis 1992; 51:152–155.

27 Petri M, Perez-Gutthann S, Spence D, Hochberg MC: Risk factors for coronary artery disease in patients with systemic lupus erythematosus. Am J Med 1992;93:513–519.

28 Manzi S, Selzer F, Sutton-Tyrrell K, Fitzgerald SG, Rairie JE, Tracy RP, Kuller LH: Prevalence and risk factors of carotid plaque in women with systemic lupus erythematosus. Arthritis Rheum 1999;42:51–60.

29 Garcia-Gomez C, Nolla JM, Valverde J, Narvaez J, Corbella E, Pinto X: High HDL-cholesterol in women with rheumatoid arthritis on low-dose glucocorticoid therapy. Eur J Clin Invest 2008;38:686–692.

30 Kuroki Y, Kaji H, Kawano S, Kanda F, Takai Y, Kajikawa M, Sugimoto T: Prospective short-term effects of glucocorticoid treatment on glucose and lipid metabolism in Japanese. Intern Med 2010;49:897–902.

31 Kishikawa H, Nishimura K, Soda T, Yamanaka K, Hirai T, Kyo M, Takeda M, Fujisawa M, Kokado Y, Ichikawa Y: Low-dose steroid maintenance for renal transplant recipients. Transplant Proc 2010;42:4030–4032.

32 Toms TE, Panoulas VF, Douglas KM, Griffiths HR, Kitas GD: Lack of association between glucocorticoid use and presence of the metabolic syndrome in patients with rheumatoid arthritis: a cross-sectional study. Arthritis Res Ther 2008;10:R145.

33 Ruyssen-Witrand A, Fautrel B, Saraux A, Le Loet X, Pham T: Cardiovascular risk induced by low-dose corticosteroids in rheumatoid arthritis: a systematic literature review. Joint Bone Spine 2011;78:23–30.

34 Davis JM 3rd, Maradit Kremers H, Crowson CS, Nicola PJ, Ballman KV, Therneau TM, Roger VL, Gabriel SE: Glucocorticoids and cardiovascular events in rheumatoid arthritis: a population-based cohort study. Arthritis Rheum 2007;56:820–830.

35 Jonsson H, Nived O, Sturfelt G: Outcome in systemic lupus erythematosus: a prospective study of patients from a defined population. Medicine (Baltimore) 1989;68:141–150.

36 Avina-Zubieta JA, Abrahamowicz M, De Vera MA, Choi HK, Sayre EC, Rahman MM, Sylvestre MP, Wynant W, Esdaile JM, Lacaille D: Immediate and past cumulative effects of oral glucocorticoids on the risk of acute myocardial infarction in rheumatoid arthritis: a population-based study. Rheumatology (Oxford) 2013;52:68–75.

37 Wei L, MacDonald TM, Walker BR: Taking glucocorticoids by prescription is associated with subsequent cardiovascular disease. Ann Intern Med 2004;141:764–770.
38 Connell JM, Whitworth JA, Davies DL, Lever AF, Richards AM, Fraser R: Effects of ACTH and cortisol administration on blood pressure, electrolyte metabolism, atrial natriuretic peptide and renal function in normal man. J Hypertens 1987;5:425–433.
39 Bia MJ, Tyler K, DeFronzo R: The effect of dexamethasone on renal potassium excretion and acute potassium tolerance. Endocrinology 1983;113:1690–1696.
40 Bia JM, Tyler K, DeFronzo RA: The effect of dexamethasone on renal electrolyte excretion in the adrenalectomized rat. Endocrinology 1982;111:882–888.
41 van Everdingen AA, Jacobs JW, Siewertsz van Reesema DR, Bijlsma JW: Low-dose prednisone therapy for patients with early active rheumatoid arthritis: clinical efficacy, disease-modifying properties, and side effects: a randomized, double-blind, placebo-controlled clinical trial. Ann Intern Med 2002;136:1–12.
42 Kirwan JR: Systemic low-dose glucocorticoid treatment in rheumatoid arthritis. Rheum Dis Clin North Am 2001;27:389–403, ix–x.
43 Jackson SH, Beevers DG, Myers K: Does long-term low-dose corticosteroid therapy cause hypertension? Clin Sci (Lond) 1981;61(suppl 7):381s–383s.
44 Wassenberg S, Rau R, Steinfeld P, Zeidler H: Very low-dose prednisolone in early rheumatoid arthritis retards radiographic progression over two years: a multicenter, double-blind, placebo-controlled trial. Arthritis Rheum 2005;52:3371–3380.
45 Capell HA, Madhok R, Hunter JA, Porter D, Morrison E, Larkin J, Thomson EA, Hampson R, Poon FW: Lack of radiological and clinical benefit over two years of low-dose prednisolone for rheumatoid arthritis: results of a randomised controlled trial. Ann Rheum Dis 2004;63:797–803.
46 Kirwan JR, Hallgren R, Mielants H, Wollheim F, Bjorck E, Persson T, Book C, Bowman S, Byron M, Cox N, Field M, Kanerud L, Leirisalo-Repo M, Malaise M, Mohammad A, Palmer R, Petersson IF, Ringertz B, Sheldon P, Simonsson M, Snowden N, Van den Bosch F: A randomised placebo controlled 12 week trial of budesonide and prednisolone in rheumatoid arthritis. Ann Rheum Dis 2004;63:688–695.
47 Kirwan JR: The effect of glucocorticoids on joint destruction in rheumatoid arthritis. The Arthritis and Rheumatism Council Low-Dose Glucocorticoid Study Group. N Engl J Med 1995;333:142–146.
48 Boers M, Verhoeven AC, Markusse HM, van de Laar MA, Westhovens R, van Denderen JC, van Zeben D, Dijkmans BA, Peeters AJ, Jacobs P, van den Brink HR, Schouten HJ, van der Heijde DM, Boonen A, van der Linden S: Randomised comparison of combined step-down prednisolone, methotrexate and sulphasalazine with sulphasalazine alone in early rheumatoid arthritis. Lancet 1997;350:309–318.
49 Pryor BD, Bologna SG, Kahl LE: Risk factors for serious infection during treatment with cyclophosphamide and high-dose corticosteroids for systemic lupus erythematosus. Arthritis Rheum 1996;39:1475–1482.
50 Greenberg JD, Reed G, Kremer JM, Tindall E, Kavanaugh A, Zheng C, Bishai W, Hochberg MC: Association of methotrexate and tumour necrosis factor antagonists with risk of infectious outcomes including opportunistic infections in the CORRONA registry. Ann Rheum Dis 2010;69:380–386.
51 Grijalva CG, Chen L, Delzell E, Baddley JW, Beukelman T, Winthrop KL, Griffin MR, Herrinton LJ, Liu L, Ouellet-Hellstrom R, Patkar NM, Solomon DH, Lewis JD, Xie F, Saag KG, Curtis JR: Initiation of tumor necrosis factor-α antagonists and the risk of hospitalization for infection in patients with autoimmune diseases. JAMA 2011;306:2331–2339.
52 Stuck AE, Minder CE, Frey FJ: Risk of infectious complications in patients taking glucocorticosteroids. Rev Infect Dis 1989;11:954–963.
53 Ruyssen-Witrand A, Fautrel B, Saraux A, Le-Loet X, Pham T: Infections induced by low-dose corticosteroids in rheumatoid arthritis: a systematic literature review. Joint Bone Spine 2010;77:246–251.
54 Svensson B, Boonen A, Albertsson K, van der Heijde D, Keller C, Hafstrom I: Low-dose prednisolone in addition to the initial disease-modifying antirheumatic drug in patients with early active rheumatoid arthritis reduces joint destruction and increases the remission rate: a two-year randomized trial. Arthritis Rheum 2005;52:3360–3370.
55 Dixon WG, Kezouh A, Bernatsky S, Suissa S: The influence of systemic glucocorticoid therapy upon the risk of non-serious infection in older patients with rheumatoid arthritis: a nested case-control study. Ann Rheum Dis 2011;70:956–960.
56 Conn HO, Blitzer BL: Nonassociation of adrenocorticosteroid therapy and peptic ulcer. N Engl J Med 1976;294:473–479.
57 Messer J, Reitman D, Sacks HS, Smith H Jr, Chalmers TC: Association of adrenocorticosteroid therapy and peptic-ulcer disease. N Engl J Med 1983;309:21–24.
58 Piper JM, Ray WA, Daugherty JR, Griffin MR: Corticosteroid use and peptic ulcer disease: role of nonsteroidal anti-inflammatory drugs. Ann Intern Med 1991;114:735–740.
59 Hernandez-Diaz S, Rodriguez LA: Association between nonsteroidal anti-inflammatory drugs and upper gastrointestinal tract bleeding/perforation: an overview of epidemiologic studies published in the 1990s. Arch Intern Med 2000;160:2093–2099.
60 Garcia Rodriguez LA, Lin KJ, Hernandez-Diaz S, Johansson S: Risk of upper gastrointestinal bleeding with low-dose acetylsalicylic acid alone and in combination with clopidogrel and other medications. Circulation 2011;123:1108–1115.
61 Conn HO, Poynard T: Corticosteroids and peptic ulcer: meta-analysis of adverse events during steroid therapy. J Intern Med 1994;236:619–632.
62 Saab S, Corr MP, Weisman MH: Corticosteroids and systemic lupus erythematosus pancreatitis: a case series. J Rheumatol 1998;25:801–806.
63 Sadr-Azodi O, Mattsson F, Bexlius TS, Lindblad M, Lagergren J, Ljung R: Association of oral glucocorticoid use with an increased risk of acute pancreatitis: a population-based nested case-control study. JAMA Intern Med 2013;173:444–449.
64 Lewis DA, Smith RE: Steroid-induced psychiatric syndromes: a report of 14 cases and a review of the literature. J Affect Disord 1983;5:319–332.
65 Drug-induced convulsions. Report from Boston Collaborative Drug Surveillance Program. Lancet 1972;2:677–679.
66 Warrington TP, Bostwick JM: Psychiatric adverse effects of corticosteroids. Mayo Clin Proc 2006;81:1361–1367.
67 Bolanos SH, Khan DA, Hanczyc M, Bauer MS, Dhanani N, Brown ES: Assessment of mood states in patients receiving long-term corticosteroid therapy and in controls with patient-rated and clinician-rated scales. Ann Allergy Asthma Immunol 2004;92:500–505.
68 Chau SY, Mok CC: Factors predictive of corticosteroid psychosis in patients with systemic lupus erythematosus. Neurology 2003;61:104–107.
69 Patten SB, Neutel CI: Corticosteroid-induced adverse psychiatric effects: incidence, diagnosis and management. Drug Saf 2000;22:111–122.
70 Sabio JM, Vargas-Hitos JA, Navarrete N, Hidalgo-Tenorio C, Jimenez-Alonso J: Effects of low or medium-dose of prednisone on insulin resistance in patients with systemic lupus erythematosus. Clin Exp Rheumatol 2010;28:483–489.
71 Gurwitz JH, Bohn RL, Glynn RJ, Monane M, Mogun H, Avorn J: Glucocorticoids and the risk for initiation of hypoglycemic therapy. Arch Intern Med 1994;154:97–101.
72 Wolverton SE: Monitoring for adverse effects from systemic drugs used in dermatology. J Am Acad Dermatol 1992;26:661–679.

73 Curtis JR, Westfall AO, Allison J, Bijlsma JW, Freeman A, George V, Kovac SH, Spettell CM, Saag KG: Population-based assessment of adverse events associated with long-term glucocorticoid use. Arthritis Rheum 2006;55:420–426.

74 Tataranni PA, Larson DE, Snitker S, Young JB, Flatt JP, Ravussin E: Effects of glucocorticoids on energy metabolism and food intake in humans. Am J Physiol 1996;271:E317–E325.

75 Pedrosa MC, Rohrer RM, Kaplan MM: Alternate-day prednisone therapy after orthotopic liver transplantation. N Engl J Med 1991;325:1658–1659.

76 Danowski TS, Bonessi JV, Sabeh G, Sutton RD, Webster MW Jr, Sarver ME: Probabilities of pituitary-adrenal responsiveness after steroid therapy. Ann Intern Med 1964;61:11–26.

77 LaRochelle GE Jr, LaRochelle AG, Ratner RE, Borenstein DG: Recovery of the hypothalamic-pituitary-adrenal (HPA) axis in patients with rheumatic diseases receiving low-dose prednisone. Am J Med 1993;95:258–264.

78 Wood JB, Frankland AW, James VH, Landon J: A rapid test of adrenocortical function. Lancet 1965;1:243–245.

79 Daly JR, Myles AB, Bacon PA, Beardwell CG, Savage O: Pituitary adrenal function during corticosteroid withdrawal in rheumatoid arthritis. Ann Rheum Dis 1967;26:18–25.

80 Kirwan JR, Hickey SH, Hallgren R, Mielants H, Bjorck E, Persson T, Wollheim FA: The effect of therapeutic glucocorticoids on the adrenal response in a randomized controlled trial in patients with rheumatoid arthritis. Arthritis Rheum 2006;54:1415–1421.

81 MacAdams MR, White RH, Chipps BE: Reduction of serum testosterone levels during chronic glucocorticoid therapy. Ann Intern Med 1986;104:648–651.

82 Hampson G, Bhargava N, Cheung J, Vaja S, Seed PT, Fogelman I: Low circulating estradiol and adrenal androgens concentrations in men on glucocorticoids: a potential contributory factor in steroid-induced osteoporosis. Metabolism 2002;51:1458–1462.

83 Davis GF: Adverse effects of corticosteroids. II. Systemic. Clin Dermatol 1986;4:161–169.

84 James ER: The etiology of steroid cataract. J Ocul Pharmacol Ther 2007;23:403–420.

85 Saag KG, Koehnke R, Caldwell JR, Brasington R, Burmeister LF, Zimmerman B, Kohler JA, Furst DE: Low-dose long-term corticosteroid therapy in rheumatoid arthritis: an analysis of serious adverse events. Am J Med 1994;96:115–123.

86 Tripathi RC, Parapuram SK, Tripathi BJ, Zhong Y, Chalam KV: Corticosteroids and glaucoma risk. Drugs Aging 1999;15:439–450.

87 Healey LA: Rheumatoid arthritis in the elderly. Clin Rheum Dis 1986;12:173–179.

NeuroImmunoModulation

Neuroimmunomodulation 2015;22:83–88
DOI: 10.1159/000362731

Published online: September 12, 2014

Hypothalamic-Pituitary-Adrenal Axis Function in Patients with Rheumatoid Arthritis Treated with Different Glucocorticoid Approaches

Rieke Alten Edgar Wiebe

Schlosspark-Klinik, Charité University Medicine Berlin, Berlin, Germany

Key Words
Hypothalamic-pituitary-adrenal axis function · Glucocorticoids · Modified-release prednisone · Rheumatoid arthritis

Abstract
Glucocorticoids (GCs) continue to be an important treatment option in rheumatoid arthritis (RA) – despite their multitude of side effects. Amongst those, suppression of the hypothalamic-pituitary-adrenal (HPA) axis plays a dominant role. In clinical practice, low-dose GC therapy of 5 mg or less per day seems to be safest in eschewing these undesirable effects and assuring function of the HPA axis. Further research has shown that, apart from dosage, the degree of HPA axis suppression by exogenous GCs is not only dependent on the duration of therapy, but that it also underlies a significant diurnal variation. The recent development of a novel modified-release (MR) prednisone formula reflects an attempt at targeting these circadian neuroendocrine pathways of the HPA axis' function and their interplay with the immune system in RA. Data from a subset of 28 patients included in the CAPRA-1 study indicated that chronotherapy with MR prednisone has no adverse effect on HPA function. Whether adapting GC therapy to a pathophysiological circadian pattern might even be beneficial will have to be further investigated. © 2014 S. Karger AG, Basel

Introduction

The groundbreaking discovery of the anti-inflammatory and immunosuppressive properties of 'Compound E' or cortisone by Hench and Kendall in 1948 marked the beginning of the ability of physicians to treat and control autoimmune diseases. Ever since, GCs have been a cornerstone in the treatment of rheumatic diseases – with treatment regimens and administration forms changing constantly in the past decades by adapting to the latest scientific findings. In fact, soon after the successful use of pharmaceutically manufactured cortisone, Hench became aware of its mineralocorticoid adverse effects – namely sodium/water retention and potassium loss [1]. Not much later, the initial enthusiasm was further dampened by a report in 1952 by Fraser et al. [2]. They reported the post-operative collapse and death of a woman who had received prednisolone for 6 months. In the postmortem analysis, an atrophy of both adrenal glands was found. Further reports accumulated showing corticosteroid-induced adrenal suppression to result in severe post-operative complications [3]. With increasing knowledge on the complications of long-term corticosteroid therapy in patients with rheumatoid arthritis (RA), the essential role of the hypothalamic-pituitary-adrenal (HPA) axis and its susceptibility to

KARGER

E-Mail karger@karger.com
www.karger.com/nim

1021–7401/14/0222–0083$39.50/0

Rieke Alten, MD
Department of Internal Medicine II
Rheumatology, Clinical Immunology and Osteology, Schlosspark-Klinik
Charité University Medicine Berlin, Heubnerweg 2, DE–14059 Berlin (Germany)
E-Mail rieke.alten@schlosspark-klinik.de

suppression by exogenous glucocorticoids (GCs) were pinpointed and the exact role and benefits of corticosteroids in the treatment of RA put under considerable debate. Against the background of GC-related adverse effects, it continues to be a major challenge to find a therapeutic regimen that minimizes the constraining side effects while guaranteeing an optimal control of symptoms and autoinflammatory processes. This article provides an overview of current knowledge on different GC treatment approaches and their effects on HPA function.

Dose-Dependent HPA Axis Function

Confronted with the adverse effects on the HPA axis, findings by Danowski et al. [4] could show that the probability of HPA axis suppression was related to the duration and dosage of GC therapy, i.e. higher doses over a longer period of time caused more pronounced suppression of the pituitary-adrenal function. In 1993, LaRochelle et al. [5] outlined a correlation between prednisone dose and HPA axis response to stimuli, favoring less than 5 mg per day for normal HPA function. These results reflected previous findings by Daly et al. [6], who, in 1967, showed that median plasma cortisol levels only remained in normal ranges in patients when receiving less than 5 mg of prednisolone per day. Yet, interestingly, in the latter study, there seemed to be no definite correlation between individual plasma cortisol levels and dose and duration of prednisolone treatment. Similarly, in 1992, Schlaghecke et al. [7] tested the degree of pituitary-adrenal function in patients treated with different doses of synthetic GC medication for different periods by measuring the pituitary-adrenal response after stimulation with corticotropin-releasing hormone (CRH). They concluded that the pituitary-adrenal function could not be estimated from dose, duration of therapy or basal plasma values of cortisol. Even EULAR recommendations on GC therapy state that 'hypothalamic-pituitary-adrenal axis suppression may vary greatly from person to person and continues to be difficult to predict' [8]. Current EULAR guidelines integrate the concept of dose-dependent HPA axis effects of GCs and underline that HPA axis suppression is likely to occur with treatment that exceeds the equivalent of 7.5 mg of prednisolone for more than 3 weeks [9].

The low-dose GC approach as an initial or maintenance therapy originated mainly from findings that showed that low-dose therapy was as effective in relieving patients from symptoms and preventing disease progression in the short and medium term, and at the same time reduced the adverse effects of long-term therapy [10–12]. Several other studies have shown that the benefit/risk ratio is favorable for low-dose therapy. Still, most recently, Kirwan et al. [13] demonstrated in a randomized, double-blind, placebo-controlled trial that in previously GC-naïve patients, 7.5 mg of prednisolone per day also suppressed HPA activity (measured after ACTH stimulation test). Thus, it seems that GC therapy and its effects on the HPA axis remains likely to also be defined by the treatment regimen, rather than dosage alone.

Targeting the Time of Day of GC Administration

In the early beginnings of systematic GC therapy of RA, different regimens were investigated in order to find a way of administering GCs effectively with the least suppression of the HPA axis. In a special report from 2011, Kirwan [14] gives a detailed overview of the historical development of how the current treatment rationale evolved in favor of targeting the time of day of GC delivery. Briefly, midnight administration of GCs was shown by Nichols et al. [15] to completely suppress cortisol production for 24 h, while giving the same dose at 8 a.m. or 4 p.m. would suppress GC secretion from the adrenal gland only transiently and less intensely. This diurnal variation indicated that HPA axis function goes beyond a simple negative feedback mechanism and represented a clear case for adapting GC therapy to the timing of the day. In addition, findings in which HPA axis suppression was shown to be more severe in multiple daily dose administration with more pronounced side effects while being less potent in controlling symptoms [16], supported the recommendation of a single morning dose regimen [17]. This concept was further substantiated by analyses by Weitzman et al. [18], who outlined the episodic secretion of cortisol, making morning doses of exogenous GCs the optimal timing in theory – just after the physiological endogenous GC peak.

However, data remained controversial, especially in regard to controlling morning symptoms, such as morning stiffness, because some patients favored a nocturnal dose of prednisolone [19, 20]. Thus, treatment options were in a somewhat stymieing situation where safety was potentially traded off against efficacy – paving the way for new treatment approaches that targeted the circadian pathophysiology of RA.

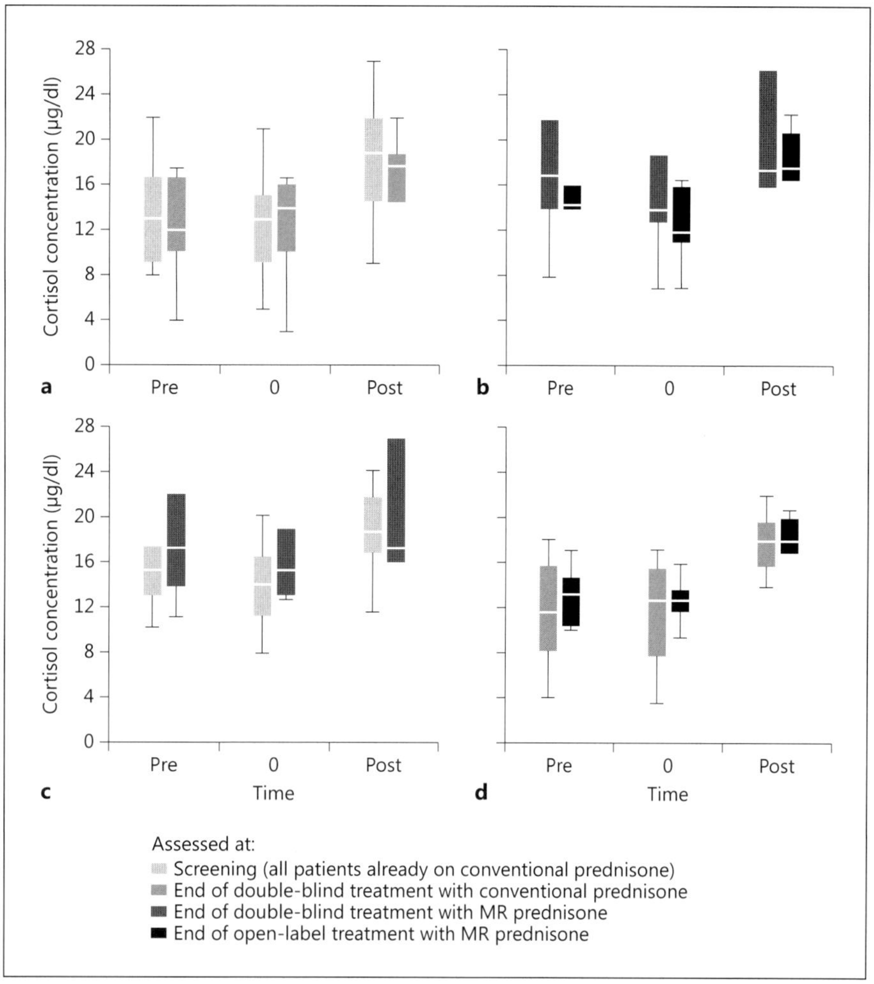

Fig. 1. Responses to CRH testing in subgroups of patients included in the CAPRA-1 study according to treatment [38]. Data are presented from assessments made 15 min before (Pre), immediately before (0) and the highest of 30 or 60 min after (Post) CRH testing. **a** Patients (n = 11) remaining on treatment with conventional prednisone. **b** Patients (n = 7) remaining on treatment with MR prednisone. **c** Patients (n = 7) switched from conventional (at screening) to MR prednisone (measure at the end of double blind phase). **d** Patients (n = 9) switched from conventional (during double blind phase) to MR prednisone (measured at the end of open-label treatment). Figure modified after Alten et al. [38].

Circadian Rhythms and HPA Axis Deficiency in Patients with RA

With recent insights into the role of endogenous and exogenous GCs [21], and a better understanding of the involvement of neuroendocrine pathways in the function of the HPA axis and their interplay with the immune system in RA [22–26], new treatment options arose. The basis was found by Arvidson et al. [27] when proposing that key symptoms such as morning stiffness in RA were likely to be attributable to circadian rhythms of plasma concentrations of IL-6 (which peaked in the morning and abated during the day).

Mastorakos et al. [28] showed in 1993 that recombinant IL-6 stimulated the HPA axis and led to a marked and prolonged elevation of plasma ACTH and cortisol levels. A plethora of studies investigating the HPA axis function of patients with RA strengthened the concept, that although the HPA axis seems to function normally in patients with RA, its defect lies in its insufficiency to react with adequately high levels of cortisol to increased inflammation [29–31].

The link between diurnal endogenous GC production and stimulation by (auto-) inflammatory cytokines formed the basis for attempting a new strategy in which this 'HPA axis insufficiency' would be tackled by administering GCs at a time point where elevated GC levels are needed the most to control rising pro-inflammatory cytokines responsible for the main symptoms, such as morning stiffness [24]. This approach, where a group of patients received low-dose prednisolone at 2 a.m. as compared to a group receiving the same dose at 7.30 a.m. proved extremely effective in reducing circadian symptoms [32].

These early findings were the cradle for the development of a preparation of a novel modified-release (MR)

Table 1. Plasma cortisol levels after stimulation with CRH [38]

Treatment and assessment time	n	Mean plasma cortisol (± SD), μg/dl	Maximum plasma cortisol, μg/dl
Conventional prednisone (pre-study)	21	5.5±4.37	15.00
Conventional prednisone (after 12 weeks double-blind phase)	11	4.5±3.91	13.85
MR prednisone (after 12 weeks double-blind phase)	8	3.3±5.76	12.00
MR prednisone (after 9 months open-label phase)	22	5.3±4.07	13.01

prednisone formulation, which, when taken at bedtime, releases the drug at around 2 a.m. prior to the rise of pro-inflammatory cytokines. In the past few years, two large studies on GC chronotherapy with MR prednisone – Administration of Prednisone in Rheumatoid Arthritis (CAPRA)-1 plus open-label extension and CAPRA-2 – have clearly shown its clinical efficacy [33–35], safety and tolerability [36–38]. Yet, although the safety profile of MR prednisone is favorable and clinically not different from conventional prednisone [37], the question was raised as to what the impact of this new formula specifically on the HPA axis might be.

Chronotherapy and Its Effect on the HPA Axis: Current Data

In the pilot study by Arvidson et al. [32], it was pointed out that from a theoretical point of view, administration of nocturnal GCs could be controversial since it does not coincide with the circadian rhythm of endogenous GC secretion. Although chronotherapy with MR prednisone represents an approach to targeting the pathophysiological pattern of the circadian neuroendocrine-immune system in RA, the exact effect on the HPA axis could not be predicted a priori. With limited knowledge on the effects of long-term night-time prednisone application, it was therefore important to assess the impact of MR prednisone on the HPA axis.

The function of the HPA axis was tested in a subset of 28 patients included in the CAPRA-1 study – for a detailed description, see Alten et al. [38]. Briefly, CRH-stimulation tests were performed at three different time points: at baseline, at 12 weeks of treatment with either conventional or MR prednisone, and after the 9-month open-label extension phase with MR prednisone. Exogenous human CRH was administered and cortisol plasma levels analyzed 15 min before, immediately before and 60 and 90 min after injection. The response to CRH was rated as either normal (52.4%), suppressed (33.3%) or no response (14.3%).

Over a period of 12 months, no deterioration or onset of adrenal insufficiency was noted. Mean cortisol response did not differ between time points (table 1; fig. 1), and the proportion of responders remained constant. Switching from conventional to MR prednisone (during the open-label phase) also did not negatively influence the response. This clearly indicated that chronotherapy with MR prednisone has no adverse effect on HPA axis function. Also, although the plasma cortisol level in this study did not change between the start and endpoint, a separate detailed study of plasma cortisol concentrations in patients treated with MR prednisone showed an enhanced nocturnal cortisol peak after 2 weeks of treatment [39]. This potential beneficial effect of chronotherapy on HPA axis function was corroborated by a within-patient analysis of the CAPRA-1 patients who, after being on conventional prednisone from baseline for the first 12 weeks, switched to MR prednisone for 9 months. The statistically significant ($p < 0.05$) 12% increase in maximum cortisol response even suggested an improved HPA axis responsiveness in RA patients with chronotherapy compared to conventional morning prednisone treatment [40].

Conclusion

Our experience with exogenous GC therapy has shown us that the effects on HPA axis function are strongly related to the respective treatment approach, including dosage, duration, disease activity and circadian rhythms. In the light of the current concept of insufficient endogenous GC secretion due to a disturbed HPA axis in RA, it seems that adapting GC therapy to a pathophysiological circadian pattern does not only reduce symptoms associated with circadian rise of pro-inflammatory cytokines, but may also possibly improve HPA function. Despite these encouraging results, further studies with larger populations and in a long-term setting are warranted to substantiate the potential beneficial effects of MR prednisone on HPA function. Regardless, it will remain a challenge to offer a GC approach that completely reduces the risk of HPA suppression. The most promising approach in this regard is future research that aims at further revealing the interplay between the neuroendocrine and immune systems – it will help us to better understand the variability in HPA function of patients undergoing GC treatment, especially in regard to GC resistance, and make GC therapy safer and more effective.

References

1 Ward E, Slocumb CH, Polley HF, Kendall EC, Hench PS: Clinical effects of cortisone administered orally to 100 patients with rheumatoid arthritis. Ann Rheum Dis 1951;10:477–484.
2 Fraser CG, Preuss FS, Bigford WD: Adrenal atrophy and irreversible shock associated with cortisone therapy. J Am Med Assoc 1952; 149:1542–1543.
3 Jasani MK, Boyle JA, Greig WR, Dalakos TG, Browning MCK, Thompson A, et al: Corticosteroid-induced suppression of the hypothalamo-pituitary-adrenal axis: observations on patients given oral corticosteroids for rheumatoid arthritis. Q J Med 1967;36:261–276.
4 Danowski TS, Bonessi JV, Sabeh G, Sutton RD, Webster MW Jr, Sarver ME: Probabilities of pituitary-adrenal responsiveness after steroid therapy. Ann Intern Med 1964;61:11–26.
5 LaRochelle GE Jr, LaRochelle AG, Ratner RE, Borenstein DG: Recovery of the hypothalamic-pituitary-adrenal (HPA) axis in patients with rheumatic diseases receiving low-dose prednisone. Am J Med 1993;95:258–264.
6 Daly JR, Myles AB, Bacon PA, Beardwell CG, Savage O: Pituitary adrenal function during corticosteroid withdrawal in rheumatoid arthritis. Ann Rheum Dis 1967;26:18–25.
7 Schlaghecke R, Kornely E, Santen RT, Ridderskamp P: The effect of long-term glucocorticoid therapy on pituitary-adrenal responses to exogenous corticotropin-releasing hormone. New Engl J Med 1992;326:226–230.
8 Duru N, van der Goes MC, Jacobs JWG, Andrews T, Boers M, Buttgereit F, et al: EULAR evidence-based and consensus-based recommendations on the management of medium to high-dose glucocorticoid therapy in rheumatic diseases. Ann Rheum Dis 2013;72: 1905–1913.
9 Hoes JN, Jacobs JWG, Boers M, Boumpas D, Buttgereit F, Caeyers N, et al: EULAR evidence-based recommendations on the management of systemic glucocorticoid therapy in rheumatic diseases. Ann Rheum Dis 2007; 66:1560–1567.
10 Bijlsma JWJ, van der Goes MC, Hoes JN, Jacobs JWG, Buttgereit F, Kirwan J: Low-dose glucocorticoid therapy in rheumatoid arthritis: an obligatory therapy. Ann NY Acad Sci 2010;1193:123–126.
11 Svensson B, Boonen A, Albertsson K, van der Heijde D, Keller C, Hafstrom I: Low-dose prednisolone in addition to the initial disease-modifying antirheumatic drug in patients with early active rheumatoid arthritis reduces joint destruction and increases the remission rate: a two-year randomized trial. Arthritis Rheum 2005;52:3360–3370.
12 Kirwan JR, Buttgereit F: Symptom control with low-dose glucocorticoid therapy for rheumatoid arthritis. Rheumatology 2012; 51(suppl 4):iv14–iv20.
13 Kirwan JR, Hickey SH, Hallgren R, Mielants H, Bjorck E, Persson T, et al: The effect of therapeutic glucocorticoids on the adrenal response in a randomized controlled trial in patients with rheumatoid arthritis. Arthritis Rheum 2006;54:1415–1421.
14 Kirwan JR: Targeting the time of day for glucocorticoid delivery in rheumatoid arthritis. Int J Clin Rheumatol 2011;6:273–279.
15 Nichols T, Nugent CA, Tyler FH: Diurnal variation in suppression of adrenal function by glucocorticoids. J Clin Endocrinol Metab 1965;25:343–349.
16 Klinefelter HF, Winkenwerder WL, Bledsoe T: Single daily dose prednisone therapy. JAMA 1979;241:2721–2723.
17 Diraimondo VC, Forsham PH: Pharmacophysiologic principles in the use of corticoids and adrenocorticotropin. Metabolism 1958;7: 5–24.
18 Weitzman ED, Fukushima D, Nogeire C, Roffwarg H, Gallagher TF, Hellman L: Twenty-four hour pattern of the episodic secretion of cortisol in normal subjects. J Clin Endocrinol Metab 1971;33:14–22.
19 Deandrade JR, McCormick JN, Hill AG: Small doses of prednisolone in the management of rheumatoid arthritis. Ann Rheum Dis 1964;23:158–162.
20 De Silva M, Binder A, Hazleman BL: The timing of prednisolone dosage and its effect on morning stiffness in rheumatoid arthritis. Ann Rheum Dis 1984;43:790–793.
21 Buttgereit F, Burmester G-R, Straub RH, Seibel MJ, Zhou H: Exogenous and endogenous glucocorticoids in rheumatic diseases. Arthritis Rheum 2011;63:1–9.
22 Cutolo M, Straub RH, Buttgereit F: Circadian rhythms of nocturnal hormones in rheumatoid arthritis: translation from bench to bedside. Ann Rheum Dis 2008;67:905–908.
23 Straub RH, Schaible HG, Wahle M, Schedlowski M, Neeck G, Buttgereit F: Neuroendocrine-immunologic mechanisms in rheumatic diseases – a congress report (in German). Z Rheumatol 2002;61:195–200.
24 Straub RH, Cutolo M: Circadian rhythms in rheumatoid arthritis: implications for pathophysiology and therapeutic management. Arthritis Rheum 2007;56:399–408.
25 Eijsbouts AM, van den Hoogen FH, Laan RF, Hermus AR, Sweep CG, van de Putte LB: Hypothalamic-pituitary-adrenal axis activity in patients with rheumatoid arthritis. Clin Exp Rheumatol 2005;23:658–664.
26 Perry MG, Kirwan JR, Jessop DS, Hunt LP: Overnight variations in cortisol, interleukin 6, tumour necrosis factor alpha and other cytokines in people with rheumatoid arthritis. Ann Rheum Dis 2009;68:63–68.
27 Arvidson NG, Gudbjornsson B, Elfman L, Ryden AC, Totterman TH, Hallgren R: Circadian rhythm of serum interleukin-6 in rheumatoid arthritis. Ann Rheum Dis 1994;53: 521–524.
28 Mastorakos G, Chrousos GP, Weber JS: Recombinant interleukin-6 activates the hypothalamic-pituitary-adrenal axis in humans. J Clin Endocrinol Metab 1993;77:1690–1694.
29 Harbuz MS, Jessop DS: Is there a defect in cortisol production in rheumatoid arthritis? Rheumatology 1999;38:298–302.
30 Harbuz MS, Korendowych E, Jessop D, Crown AL, Lightman SL, Kirwan JR: Hypothalamo-pituitary-adrenal axis dysregulation in patients with rheumatoid arthritis after the dexamethasone/corticotrophin releasing factor test. J Endocrinol 2003;178:55–60.
31 Cutolo M, Villaggio B, Otsa K, Aakre O, Sulli A, Seriolo B: Altered circadian rhythms in rheumatoid arthritis patients play a role in the disease's symptoms. Autoimmun Rev 2005;4: 497–502.
32 Arvidson NG, Gudbjörnsson B, Larsson A, Hällgren R: The timing of glucocorticoid administration in rheumatoid arthritis. Ann Rheum Dis 1997;56:27–31.

33 Alten R: Chronotherapy with modified-release prednisone in patients with rheumatoid arthritis. Expert Rev Clin Immunol 2012;8: 123–133.
34 Buttgereit F, Doering G, Schaeffler A, Witte S, Sierakowski S, Gromnica-Ihle E, et al: Efficacy of modified-release versus standard prednisone to reduce duration of morning stiffness of the joints in rheumatoid arthritis (CAPRA-1): a double-blind, randomised controlled trial. Lancet 2008;371:205–214.
35 Buttgereit F, Doering G, Schaeffler A, Witte S, Sierakowski S, Gromnica-Ihle E, et al: Targeting pathophysiological rhythms: prednisone chronotherapy shows sustained efficacy in rheumatoid arthritis. Ann Rheum Dis 2010; 69:1275–1280.
36 Buttgereit F, Mehta DP, Kirwan JR, Szechinski J, Boers M, Alten R: Safety data for low-dose glucocorticoid chronotherapy of rheumatoid arthritis with 5 mg modified-release (MR) prednisone in a randomized, double-blind placebo-controlled trial. Ann Rheum Dis 2010;63(suppl 3):219.
37 Buttgereit F, Szechinski J, Doering G, Witte S, Knauer C, Grahn A: Integrated summary of safety for modified-release prednisone compraed to immediate release prednisone: results from the Circadian Administration of Prednisone in Rheumatoid Arthritis (CAPRA) studies. Ann Rheum Dis 2011;70(suppl 3):88.
38 Alten R, Doring G, Cutolo M, Gromnica-Ihle E, Witte S, Straub R, et al: Hypothalamus-pituitary-adrenal axis function in patients with rheumatoid arthritis treated with nighttime-release prednisone. J Rheumatol 2010;37: 2025–2031.
39 Kirwan JR, Clarke L, Hunt LP, Perry MG, Straub RH, Jessop DS: Effect of novel therapeutic glucocorticoids on circadian rhythms of hormones and cytokines in rheumatoid arthritis. Ann NY Acad Sci 2010;1193:127–133.
40 Kirwan JR: Targeting the time of day for glucocorticoid delivery in rheumatoid arthritis. Int J Clin Rheumatol 2011;6:273–279.

NeuroImmunoModulation

Neuroimmunomodulation 2015;22:89–103
DOI: 10.1159/000362735

Published online: September 12, 2014

The Past versus the Present, 1980–2004: Reduction of Mean Initial Low-Dose, Long-Term Glucocorticoid Therapy in Rheumatoid Arthritis from 10.3 to 3.6 mg/Day, Concomitant with Early Methotrexate, with Long-Term Effectiveness and Safety of Less than 5 mg/Day

Theodore Pincus[a] Tuulikki Sokka[b] Maurizio Cutolo[c]

[a]Rush University, Medical Center, Chicago, Ill., USA; [b]Jyväskylä Central Hospital, Jyväskylä, Finland; [c]Research Laboratory and Academic Division of Clinical Rheumatology, Department of Internal Medicine, University of Genoa, Genoa, Italy

Key Words

Low-dose prednisone · Rheumatoid arthritis · Multidimensional health assessment questionnaire

Abstract

Quantitative observations are presented concerning treatment with glucocorticoids of 308 patients with rheumatoid arthritis (RA) at a weekly academic rheumatology setting over 25 years from 1980 to 2004. A database of all visits included medications and multidimensional health assessment questionnaire scores for physical function, pain and routine assessment of patient index data (RAPID3; and a surrogate RAPID3-EST), completed by each patient at each visit in routine care. Over the 5-year periods of 1980–1984, 1985–1989, 1990–1994, 1995–1999 and 2000–2004, the mean initial prednisone daily dose declined from 10.3 to 6.5, 5.1, 4.1 and 3.6 mg/day, as initial doses were >5 mg/day in 49, 16, 7, 7 and 3% of patients, 5 mg/day in 51, 80, 70, 26 and 10%, and <5 mg/day in 0, 4, 23, 67 and 86%. Reduction of prednisone doses in the respective five-year periods was accompanied by increased and earlier use of methotrexate as the first disease-modifying antirheumatic drug (DMARD) in 10, 26, 57, 71 and 78%, and methotrexate treatment in 10, 26, 74, 82 and 92% of patients within the first year of disease. Higher methotrexate doses in the respective five-year periods were used after 1990, along with lower prednisone doses. Most patients were treated indefinitely with both low-dose prednisone and methotrexate; 80% continued both medications for more than 5 years. The primary adverse events were skin-thinning and bruising. New hypertension, diabetes and cataracts were seen in fewer than 10% of patients. While efficacy and safety cannot be analyzed definitively from observational data, the data suggest that many patients with RA might be treated effectively with weekly low-dose methotrexate along with initial and long-term, low-dose prednisone of <5 mg/day.

KARGER

E-Mail karger@karger.com
www.karger.com/nim

1021–7401/14/0222–0089$39.50/0

Theodore Pincus, MD
Rush University
Medical Center
Chicago, IL 60612 (USA)
E-Mail tedpincus@gmail.com

Introduction

Glucocorticoids for the treatment of rheumatoid arthritis (RA) were documented to provide dramatic clinical improvement in 1949 [1], leading to the award of the Nobel Prize for Medicine to Hench, Kendall and Reichstein in 1950 [2]. Disease-modifying activity of moderate doses of glucocorticoids was documented during the 1950s [3]. Although the Mayo Clinic group that reported the clinical value of glucocorticoids recommended doses of cortisone equivalent to 5–10 mg/day of prednisone in 1955 [4], many patients were treated with doses of 20–60 mg/day of prednisone or prednisolone, leading to severe adverse effects in most patients [5, 6]. Therefore, in the mid-1950s, systemic glucocorticoids were recommended in RA only for acute severe disease flares or life-threatening vasculitis, or as 'bridging therapy' while awaiting the anticipated benefits of DMARDs. This approach remains standard in most textbooks and rheumatology recommendations, as seen in recent EULAR guidelines for the management of RA patients with glucocorticoids [7]. Even the most recent revision states that 'low-dose glucocorticoids should be considered as part of the initial treatment strategy (in combination with one or more DMARDs) for up to 6 months, but should be tapered as rapidly as clinically feasible' [8].

Despite guidelines and teachings over many years to limit or refrain entirely from glucocorticoids in RA, prednisone or prednisolone is taken quite commonly by many patients in many usual-care rheumatology clinical settings. For example, in the international Quantitative Standard Monitoring of Patients with RA (QUEST-RA) database in 2007, among 4,363 RA patients seen in usual care at 48 clinical sites (~100 patients per site) in 15 countries, 66% of patients had ever taken glucocorticoids, including more than 70% in Argentina, Finland, France, Ireland, Serbia and the USA, and more than 50% in 7 other countries – all but Denmark (43%) and the Netherlands (26%) [9] (table 1). An analysis of the same database in 2009 found that among 6,004 RA patients seen in usual care at 70 clinical sites in 25 countries, 49% of patients were currently taking glucocorticoids [10] (data not shown). Although the data are not from a random sample of practices in these countries, consistent patterns were found among 3 practices within each country, suggesting that the information is at least moderately generalizable.

A reassessment of glucocorticoids in RA began during the 1980s [11], contemporaneous with recognition of severe long-term outcomes of RA such as frequent work disability [12, 13], radiographic progression [14] and premature mortality [13] in many patients. A 24-week non-

Table 1. The use of DMARDs in the QUEST-RA countries reported in 2007

Country	Median delay to initiation of DMARDs, months	Mean DMARD exposure, years	Selected DMARDs ever taken: patients in the QUEST-RA study per country, %					
			prednisone	MTX	HCQ	SSZ	LEF	Any biologic agent
Denmark	10	7.9	43	85	39	64	11	23
Finland	7	14.4	74	85	**74**	**84**	21	17
France	8	9.9	83	86	55	49	**42**	**53**
Germany	15	8.4	54	78	30	36	25	29
Ireland	11	6.3	71	**92**	*15*	33	24	41
Italy	9	7.1	69	79	42	14	31	26
The Netherlands	5	8.1	*26*	91	28	35	6	19
Poland	4	7.2	69	87	34	60	18	8
Spain	14	7.3	67	82	43	29	34	27
Sweden	12	8.8	66	83	34	62	9	31
UK	12	7.9	51	*67*	39	46	*4*	16
Turkey	12	8.9	69	88	27	61	22	7
Serbia	11	6.6	**88**	69	55	17	7	*2*
USA	9	7.9	77	85	49	12	19	33
Argentina	13	3.7	83	68	49	6	16	3
Total	9	8.1	66	83	41	43	21	23

The highest percentage for each drug is highlighted in bold, and the lowest in italics. Source: Sokka et al. [9]. MTX = Methotrexate; HCQ = hydroxychloroquine; SSZ = sulfasalazine; LEF = leflunomide.

blinded clinical trial of low-dose prednisone at 5 mg/day indicated efficacy to improve clinical status and slow radiographic progression [11]. Since 1995, 10 further double-blind clinical trials [15–24] have provided strong evidence for the efficacy and safety of doses of 10 mg/day or less of prednisone in RA compared to placebo [see the article by Rasch et al.; this issue, pp. 51–56; and the article by Jacobs et al.; this issue, pp. 66–71]. Most of these clinical trials were focused on reduction of structural damage (radiographic progression) [15–19, 23, 25], and a few on functional status [11, 15]. One withdrawal trial documented clinical efficacy of 3 mg/day, a dose which patients could distinguish from placebo [21]. Reports indicating disease modification with low doses of prednisone or prednisolone of 5 mg/day [15, 19] are of particular interest, as 5 mg/day is associated with the absence of suppression of the hypothalamic-pituitary-adrenal axis [26–29], while 10 mg/day over long periods is associated with adverse effects in many patients [30], including cardiovascular disease [31], bone loss [32] and higher mortality rates [33, 34].

The 1980s also were characterized by the introduction of widespread use of methotrexate [35], which had been used by only a few practitioners to treat RA in the 1960s and 1970s [36]. Methotrexate was documented to be efficacious in clinical trials [37], and provided considerably greater long-term effectiveness, as well as considerably greater safety, than parenteral gold salts or penicillamine, which were the traditional DMARDs used until the 1980s [38]. Over the 1990s and 2000s, methotrexate was used in increasing doses earlier in the disease course. Methotrexate has become the most widely-used 'anchor drug' for RA [39], taken by 83% of patients in QUEST-RA [9], and continued for more than 5 years by more than 80% of patients of the senior author (T.P.) [40]. These developments are reflected in changes toward treatment of most RA patients with low-dose prednisone of ≤5 mg/day [41, 42] and early weekly low-dose methotrexate [43].

This article summarizes the experience of T.P. in treating RA patients with prednisone [41, 42] and methotrexate [43] over 25 years between 1980 and 2004 at a weekly academic clinical setting. A database was maintained of all visits of all patients over this period, which included medications as well as scores for functional status and pain on a multidimensional health assessment questionnaire (MDHAQ) [44–46]. Routine assessment of patient index data (RAPID3) [47]. The MDHAQ also includes self-report of possible adverse effects in each patient.

Of course, the ideal approach to evaluate the efficacy (short-term), effectiveness (long-term) and safety of any therapy is regarded to be a randomized controlled clinical trial, rather than observational data, to provide what is widely designated as 'evidence-based medicine' [48]. However, clinical trials are affected severely by many limitations, including patient selection, a short time frame, inflexible dosages, restrictions, concomitant medications, etc., which compromise the applicability to usual clinical care [49–55]. Furthermore, randomization cannot be maintained for longer than 2 years (or even 2 months) in symptomatic individuals. Therefore, long-term observational studies are needed to complement data from randomized trials [54–57]. Long-term observational data are also affected by limitations (as is true of any method used in clinical research), primarily 'confounding by indication' [58, 59], i.e. people with more severe clinical status are more likely to be treated with stronger medications and higher doses of these medications, leading to more adverse events.

Randomized controlled clinical trials and observational studies may be viewed as complementary methods, each with strengths and limitations. A recent report [60] of the Oxford Centre for Evidence-Based Medicine (OCEBM) concerning levels of evidence noted that: 'While they are simple and easy to use, early hierarchies that placed randomized trials categorically above observational studies were criticized [61] for being simplistic [62]. In some cases, observational studies give us the "best" evidence [61]. For example, there is a growing recognition that observational studies – even case-series [63] and anecdotes [64] – can sometimes provide definitive evidence' [60]. The data presented in this article are viewed as complementary to articles in this special issue by Rasch, Jacobs, Da Silva and ourselves concerning randomized controlled clinical trials involving prednisone.

This review presents evidence concerning:

(1) reduction of mean initial prednisone dose from 10.3 mg/day in 1980–1985 to 3.6 mg/day in 2000–2004, with 86% of patients seen in 2000–2004 having initial doses <5 mg/day;

(2) higher mean initial prednisone doses in patients with higher scores for MDHAQ physical function, pain and RAPID3, reflecting 'confounding by indication';

(3) increased and earlier use of methotrexate over the 25-year period, concomitant with decreased doses of prednisone, with methotrexate as the first DMARD at the first visit in 78% of patients in 2000–2004 compared to 10% in 1980–1985;

(4) similar improvement over 12 months according to MDHAQ/RAPID3 scores in patients whose initial dose was less than, equal to, or greater than 5 mg/day;

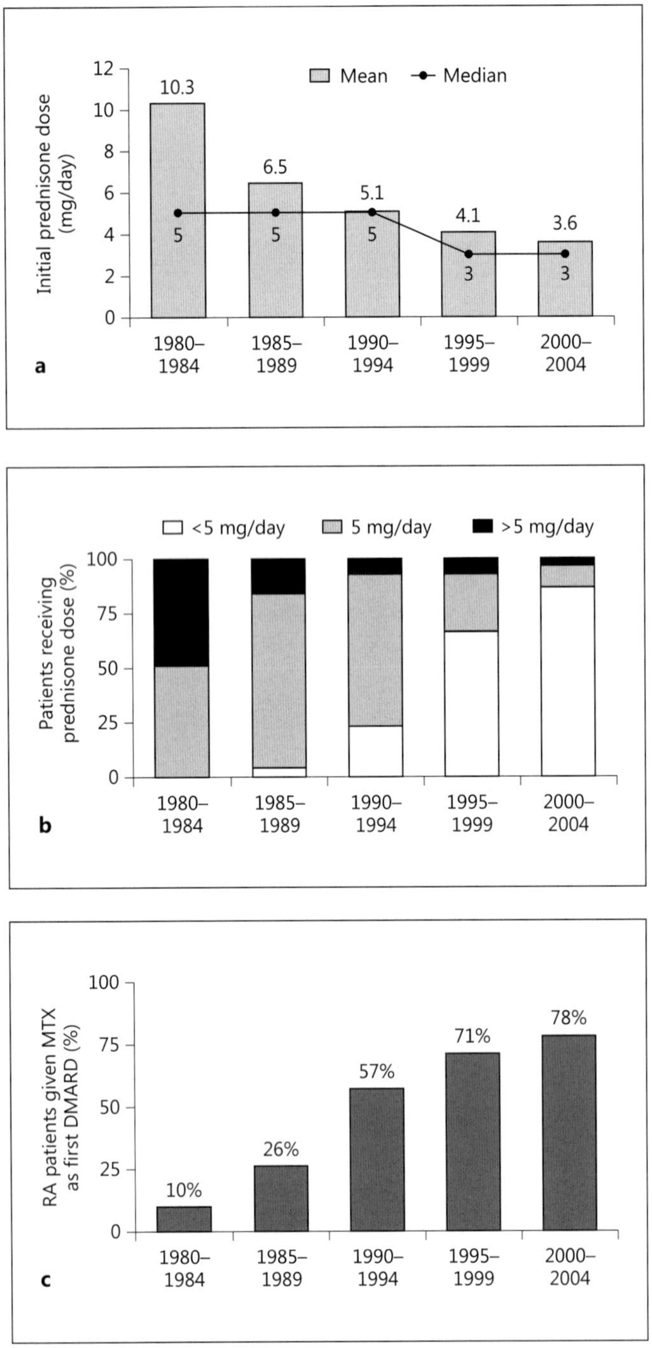

Fig. 1. a Mean and median initial prednisone dose in 308 patients with RA seen between 1980 and 2004, computed in 5-year periods: 1980–1984, 1985–1989, 1990–1994, 1995–1999 and 2000–2004. **b** Percentage of patients with RA whose initial prednisone dose was <5, 5 or >5 mg/day in the respective 5-year periods. **c** Percentage of patients with RA who were treated with methotrexate (MTX) as the initial DMARD in the respective 5-year periods [data from 43]. Source: Pincus et al. [42].

Table 2. Initial prednisone dose in 308 patients with RA seen from 1980 through to 2004

Year first seen	Patients, n	Mean initial dose, mg/day	Patients taking initial dose, %		
			<5 mg/day	5 mg/day	>5 mg/day
1980–1984	37	10.3 (5)	0	51	49
1985–1989	74	6.5 (5)	4	80	16
1990–1994	77	5.1 (5)	23	70	7
1995–1999	61	4.1 (3)	67	26	7
2000–2004	59	3.6 (3)	86	10	3

Median values are given in parentheses. Adapted from Pincus et al. [42].

(5) maintenance of improved long-term outcomes in patients treated with low-dose (<5 mg/day) prednisone over long periods, including 73 patients over more than 8 years;

(6) substantially better clinical status in all RA patients seen in this setting in 2000 versus 1985 associated with long-term low-dose prednisone;

(7) few adverse events in patients treated with low-dose (<5 mg/day) prednisone over 5–15 years, including in 73 patients treated with prednisone for longer than 8 years.

These topics are summarized below.

Decline of Mean Initial Prednisone Dose from 10.3 mg/Day in 1980–1985 to 3.6 mg/Day in 2000–2004

The initial prednisone dose in 308 patients with RA treated between 1980 and 2004 was analyzed in 5-year periods: 1980–1984, 1985–1989, 1990–1994, 1995–1999 and 2000–2004 [42] (table 2). The mean initial prednisone dose was 10.3 mg/day in 1980–1984 and fell in each 5-year period to 6.5 in 1985–1989, 5.1 in 1990–1994, 4.1 in 1995–1999 and 3.6 mg/day in 2000–2004 (table 2). The proportion treated initially with >5 mg/day was 49, 16, 7, 7 and 3% in the respective 5-year periods, compared to 51, 80, 70, 26 and 10% treated initially with 5 mg/day, and 0, 4, 23, 67 and 86% with <5 mg/day (table 2). These data indicate a reduction of more than 60% in the initial dose over the 25-year period [42].

Higher Mean Initial Prednisone Doses in Patients with Higher MDHAQ Scores

A version of an MDHAQ [45, 46] was completed by every patient at every visit. The MDHAQ includes the 3 self-report measures in the RA core data set – physical function, pain and patient estimate of global status. RAP-

Table 3. Baseline and endpoint (12-month) scores on MDHAQ for physical function and pain in 308 patients with RA, according to initial prednisone dose <5 versus ≥5 mg/day in 5-year periods between 1980 and 2004

Year first seen	Mean initial dose, mg/day	Initial dose <5 mg/day					Initial dose ≥5 mg/day				
		n	MDHAQ-function		MDHAQ-pain		n	MDHAQ-function		MDHAQ-pain	
			baseline	12 months	baseline	12 months		baseline	12 months	baseline	12 months
1980–1984	10.3 (5)	0	–	–	–	–	37	4.1	2.7	6.4	4.8
1985–1989	6.5 (5)	3	1.4	1.5	5.3	5.7	71	3.3	1.8	6.3	3.7
1990–1994	5.1 (5)	18	1.7	1.3	4.7	2.7	59	3.2	1.8	5.9	3.3
1995–1999	4.1 (3)	41	2.7	1.8	4.6	3.2	20	3.9	2.9	6.3	5.1
2000–2004	3.6 (3)	51	2.6	1.6	5.9	3.5	8	4.3	3.2	7.0	5.3
Total	5.6 (5)	113	2.4	1.6	5.2	3.3	195	3.5	2.1	6.3	4.0

Median values are given in parentheses. Source: Pincus et al. [42].

ID3, an index of these 3 patient-reported Core Data Set measures without a formal joint count, was also calculated.

Patient global estimate was not included prior to 1996. Therefore, RAPID3 was estimated as 'RAPID3-EST', a composite of 2 measures of physical function score plus pain score multiplied by 2, without a patient global estimate score [41, 42]. RAPID3-EST is correlated with RAPID3 scores at rho = 0.85 in patients in this database in whom standard RAPID3 scores were available.

Mean baseline MDHAQ physical function scores were 0.8 on a 0–3 scale and 2.4 on a 0–10 scale (recoded from 0–3 to 0–10) in patients initially treated with less than 5 mg/day, and 3.5 on a 0–10 scale (1.2 on a 0–3 scale) in patients initially treated with greater than 5 mg/day (maximum 20 mg/day; table 3; fig. 1) [42]. Mean pain scores were 5.2 (on a scale of 0–10) in patients treated initially with <5 mg/day, and 6.3 in patients treated with ≥5 mg/day (table 3; fig. 1). In patients treated initially with <5 mg/day versus those treated with ≥5 mg/day, mean RAPID3-EST was 12.4 versus 15.9 (on a scale of 0–30), and for patients for whom the full RAPID3 was available, 13.2 versus 17.3 (on a scale of 0–30; data not shown). These data indicate that patients with a more severe clinical status were more likely to be treated with higher doses of prednisone >5 mg/day [58] – i.e. 'confounding by indication' – but rarely with >10 mg/day [42].

Increased and Earlier Use of Methotrexate over the 25-Year Period, with Methotrexate as First DMARD at First Visit in 78% of Patients in 2000–2004

The RA patients seen between 1980 and 2004 were also analyzed for the proportion taking methotrexate, the interval from presentation to methotrexate prescription, and radiographic and functional status outcomes [43]. Overall, 738 consecutive patients were seen (only 308 had prednisone initiated by T.P. to be included in the analyses of prednisone therapy [41, 42], as more than half the patients were already taking prednisone at their first visit).

The reduction in prednisone dosage was associated with a reciprocal rise in methotrexate use (fig. 1c, 2) [42]. The probability of initiating methotrexate as the first DMARD over the 5-year periods was 10% in 1980–1984, 26% in 1985–1989, 57% in 1990–1994, 71% in 1995–1999 and 78% in 2000–2004 (fig. 1c) [43]. The median interval from presentation to methotrexate initiation was 8.6 years in 1980–1984, 4.4 years in 1985–1989 and <2 months in 1990–1994, 1995–1999 and 2000–2004 (fig. 2) [43].

Patient outcomes were substantially improved over the 25 years, as mean scores for physical function (on a 0–3 scale) were 1.13 in 1980–1984 versus 0.57 in 2000–2004 (or 3.4 vs. 1.7 on a 0–10 scale; fig. 3) [43]. Similar analyses in Jyväskylä, Finland, indicated that mean 5-year Larsen radiographic scores (0–100 scale) were 15.7 in 1980–1984 versus 4.0 in 1995–1999 [43]. Therefore, early methotrexate in usual clinical care of RA increased from <5% in 1980 to >75% in 2004. Substantially improved outcomes were seen over this period, most of which antedated biological agents, as these agents were introduced in 1999.

Similar Improvement in Clinical Status over 12 Months in Patients Treated with <5 mg/Day versus ≥5 mg/Day of Prednisone

Mean changes over the first 12 months of prednisone therapy were computed for MDHAQ scores for physical function, pain and RAPID3-EST in all 308 patients treat-

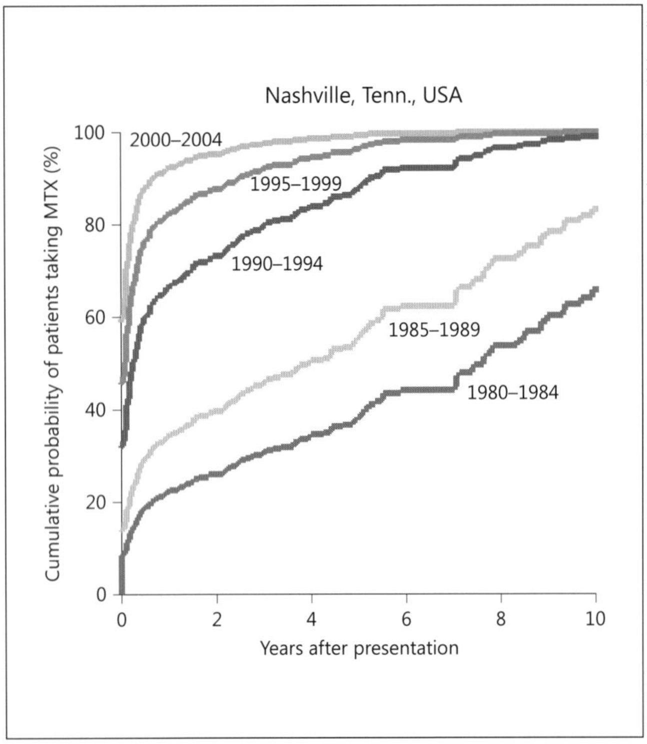

Fig. 2. Interval between patient presentation and initiation of methotrexate (MTX) in the senior author's practice in Nashville, Tenn., USA, according to the period of patient presentation. Source: Sokka and Pincus [43].

Color version available online

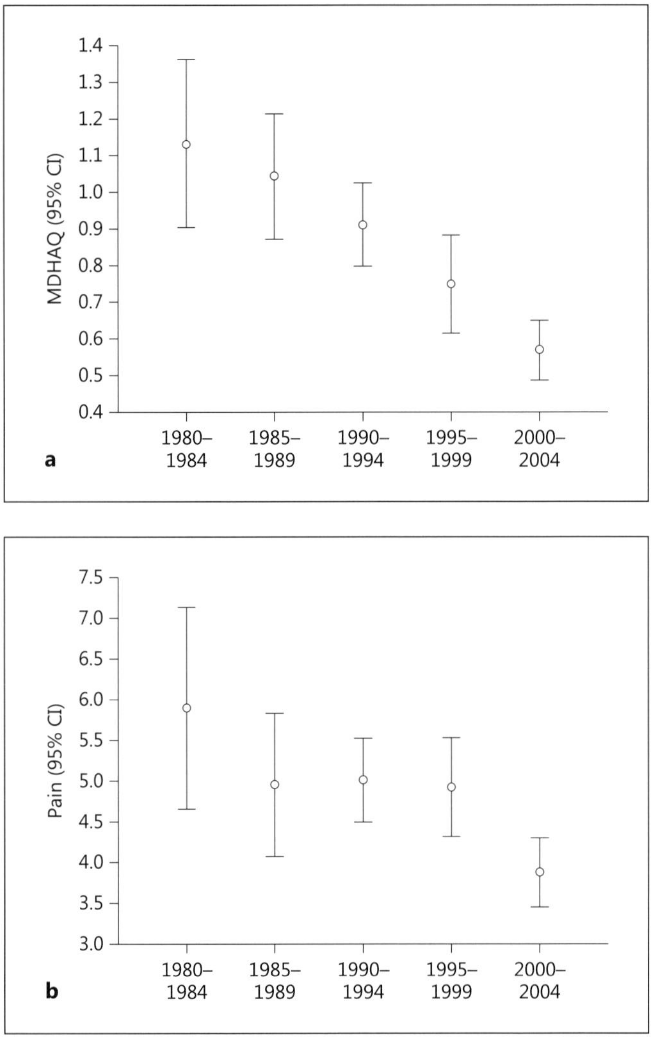

Fig. 3. Patient functional status according to MDHAQ function (**a**) and pain (**b**), in 596 patients in Nashville, Tenn., USA, at final visit, according to the period in which the last visit occurred. Source: Sokka and Pincus [43].

ed from 1980 to 2004 for whom data 1 year later were available (tables 3, 4; fig. 1) [42]. Changes were compared in patients treated with <5 versus ≥5 mg/day, as few patients received >5 mg/day [42].

In patients whose initial prednisone dose was ≥5 mg/day, scores for function, pain and RAPID3-EST fell by 40, 37 and 38%, respectively, over the subsequent 12 months (tables 3, 4; fig. 1). In patients whose initial dose was <5 mg/day, scores for function, pain and RAPID3-EST fell similarly, by 34, 37 and 37% over the subsequent 12 months [42].

The reduction in prednisone dose was associated with a reciprocal rise in the use of methotrexate, as noted, which increased as the initial DMARD from 10% of patients in 1980–1984 to 78% of patients in 2000–2004 (fig. 1c) [42, 43]. As noted (several times) below, it is impossible to separate the possible effects of methotrexate versus prednisone on reduction of functional disability and radiographic progression. Most likely, both agents were active.

Maintenance of Improved Long-Term Outcomes in Patients Treated with Low-Dose (<5 mg/Day) Prednisone over Long Periods

Mean prednisone doses appeared to be largely unchanged in patients monitored over ≤1, 1.1–4.0, 4.1–8.0 and >8 years, representing quartiles of all patients (table 5). Clinical improvement was maintained for up to 8 years in most patients (table 5) [42], although some worsening in physical function was seen in patients with the longest follow-up, consistent with aging. These findings differ considerably from those in the 1980s and 1990s, when severe declines began after 2–3 years in most patients [13, 65].

Table 4. Percentage changes in scores on MDHAQ for physical function, pain and RAPID3-EST over 12 months in 308 patients according to initial prednisone dose <5 versus ≥5 mg/day between 1980 and 2004

Year first seen	Mean initial dose, mg/day	Clinical change over 12 months, %							
		initial dose <5 mg/day				initial dose ≥5 mg/day			
		n	function	pain	RAPID3-EST	n	function	pain	RAPID3-EST
1980–1984	10.3 (5)	0	–	–	–	37	+33	+25	+28
1985–1989	6.5 (5)	3	–5	–8	–24	71	+45	+42	+43
1990–1994	5.1 (5)	18	+26	+43	+38	59	+44	+44	+42
1995–1999	4.1 (3)	41	+33	+30	+37	20	+27	+19	+25
2000–2004	3.6 (3)	51	+37	+41	+39	8	+25	+25	+30
Total	5.6 (5)	113	+34	+37	+37	195	+40	+37	+38

Median values are given in parentheses. '+' indicates improvement and '–' worsening in function, pain and RAPID3-EST scores. Adapted from Pincus et al. [42].

Table 5. Baseline and last available prednisone dose, scores on MDHAQ for physical function, pain and RAPID3-EST, and new adverse events reported by patients, according to length of prednisone treatment in 344 patients with RA

	Duration of prednisone use					Total (n = 334)
	No follow-up (n = 44)	0.1–10 years (n = 72)	1.1–4.0 years (n = 70)	4.1–8.0 years (n = 75)	>8 years (n = 73)	
Clinical MDHAQ variables, mean						
Baseline MDHAQ-function (0–10 scale)	3.4 (2.0)	3.2 (2.0)	2.8 (1.6)	3.0 (2.1)	3.3 (1.9)	3.1 (2.0)
Last visit MDHAQ-function (0–10 scale)	–	2.7 (2.3)	2.3 (1.8)	2.7 (2.3)	3.3 (2.4)	2.8 (2.2)
Baseline MDHAQ-pain (0–10 scale)	5.8 (2.8)	5.9 (2.5)	5.8 (2.6)	6.1 (2.4)	5.9 (2.6)	5.9 (2.6)
Last visit MDHAQ-pain (0–10 scale)	–	4.0 (3.0)	4.0 (2.7)	4.1 (3.0)	4.5 (3.2)	4.2 (3.0)
Baseline RAPID3-EST (0–30 scale)	14.8 (6.7)	15.1 (6.4)	14.4 (5.9)	15.0 (6.6)	14.9 (6.6)	14.8 (6.3)
Last visit RAPID3-EST (0–30 scale)	–	10.6 (7.8)	10.3 (6.7)	10.9 (7.6)	12.3 (7.9)	11.0 (7.5)
Possible adverse events						
Mean baseline weight, lb	177.0 (51.8)	163.3 (39.1)	167.3 (40.0)	161.5 (36.7)	163.5 (38.8)	165.7 (40.7)
Mean last visit weight, lb	–	169.8 (36.4)	165.6 (38.6)	160.0 (42.4)	161.4 (41.2)	164.2 (39.7)
Hypertension, n	–	1 (1.4%)	4 (5.7%)	5 (6.7%)	9 (12.3%)	19 (6.6%)
Cataracts, n	–	0	1 (1.4%)	0	8 (11.0%)	9 (3.1%)
Diabetes, n	–	0	0	3 (4.0%)	5 (6.9%)	8 (2.8%)

Mean values are given with standard deviation in parentheses; median values are given with interquartile range in parentheses. Adapted from Pincus et al. [42].

Substantially Better Clinical Status in All RA Patients Seen in 2000 versus 1985

A systematic comparison of all RA patients seen by T.P. in 1985 versus 2000 (many of whom are included in the above analyses) indicated substantially better status in 2000 according to many quantitative measures, including MDHAQ function (median score on a 0–3 scale of 1.0 vs. 0.4), swollen joint count (median 12 vs. 5), erythrocyte sedimentation rate (ESR; median 33 vs. 20 mm/h), DAS28 (5.7 vs. 4.4) and radiographic Larsen scores (median 20 vs. 3% of maximum) [66] (table 6). Most patients who did not have a positive test for rheumatoid factor had no radiographic progression at all [66]. In 1985, 51% of patients were taking prednisone with a mean daily dose of

Neuroimmunomodulation 2015;22:89–103
DOI: 10.1159/000362735

Table 6. Therapy variables and clinical status measures in two cohorts of all patients with RA seen by T.P. in 1984–1986 ('1985') versus 1999–2001 ('2000')

Variable	Cohort	
	1985	2000
Patients, n	125	150
Therapy variables		
Prednisone + any other drug, %	51	86
Mean daily dose, mg	7.8	4.6
Median daily dose, mg	5	4
Minimum daily dose, mg	4	1
Maximum daily dose, mg	30	15
Methotrexate + any other drug, %	10.4	76.7
No DMARDs, no prednisone, %	36.8	3.3
Clinical status variables		
Swollen joint count (0–28)	12 (6, 16)	5 (2, 10)
Larsen radiographic score (0–100)	20 (2, 36)	3 (0, 13)
ESR, mm/h	33 (16, 50)	20 (9, 33)
Functional disability score on MHAQ (0–3)	1.0 (0.6, 1.4)	0.4 (0.1, 1.0)
DAS28 (0–10)	5.7 (4.9, 6.5)	4.4 (3.2, 5.3)

Clinical status values depict unadjusted median values and interquartile range. p values derived from a median regression model adjusted for age, education, duration of disease and rheumatoid factor status all <0.01. Source: Pincus et al. [66].

7.8 mg/day (many patients had higher doses initiated by other physicians), 10% were taking methotrexate, and 37% no DMARDs or prednisone. In 2000, 86% were taking prednisone at a mean dose of 4.6 mg/day, 77% were taking methotrexate, and only 3% were taking no DMARDs or prednisone [66] (table 6).

These findings suggest better control of RA associated with long-term, low-dose prednisone. However, as noted, almost all patients took methotrexate and/or other DMARDs according to a policy of tight control [67, 68], particularly after 1990. Therefore, as noted, it is not possible to separate the possible effectiveness of prednisone versus methotrexate (or even, in part, a possible secular trend to milder RA [69–72]), as the data are not from a clinical trial to isolate a single variable. Nonetheless, the data, while not definitive, are consistent with clinical trial data indicating that improved outcomes are associated with low-dose prednisone, here on a long-term basis.

Few Adverse Events in Patients Treated with Low-Dose (<5 mg/Day) Prednisone over Long Periods

Adverse events were ascertained on the MDHAQ through self-report in usual care [42]. The primary adverse event was bruising and skin thinning. In 109 patients treated after 1995, the proportion of patients with hypertension was 25%, diabetes 8% and cataracts 9% (table 7) [42]. There were 6 new cases of hypertension over a mean of 5.2 years in 88 patients over 557 patient years, 5 new cases of diabetes over a mean of 5.0 years in 105 patients over 632 patient years, and 4 new cases of cataracts over a mean of 2.5 years in 103 patients over 617 patient years (table 7) [42]. The mean weight gain was 1.45 kg (median 1.13) over 48 weeks. Weight gain was lowest in patients who began prednisone ≤3 mg/day (mean 0.44 kg), and greatest in patients who began prednisone >5 mg/day (mean 2.63 kg; table 7) [42].

A formal review by a health professional might have revealed higher levels of adverse events. Nonetheless, development of diabetes, hypertension and cataracts in fewer than 10% of patients is consistent with findings in other studies [73], indicating few adverse events. It is impossible to ascertain 'expected' data for the prevalence of various comorbidities over long periods in RA patients. This level, even if 50% higher, is little or no more than would be expected in the age-matched general population.

Discussion

Observational Data in Consecutive Patients versus Randomized Controlled Clinical Trials

Assessment of the efficacy (short-term), effectiveness (long-term) and adverse events of prednisone, as well as

Table 7. Proportion of 109 RA patients who took long-term, low-dose prednisone who developed hypertension, diabetes and cataracts

Comorbidity	At baseline, n	Overall, n	New cases, n	Patient years at risk
Hypertension	21 (19%)	27 (25%)	6 (5.2)	557
Diabetes	4 (4%)	9 (8%)	5 (5.0)	632
Cataracts	6 (6%)	10 (9%)	4 (2.5)	617

Values in parentheses are either percentages, as indicated, or mean number of years. Source: Pincus et al. [42].

methotrexate, in this review article of care over 25 years is based on long-term observational data in consecutive patients rather than on data from randomized clinical trials. Observational data are affected by many limitations, primarily based on 'confounding by indication' [58, 59], i.e. that patients who have more severe disease are more likely to receive certain therapies or higher doses of such therapies, leading to more adverse events. Indeed, this possibility was documented in the reported series (table 3) [42], as higher doses of prednisone were prescribed for patients who had a more severe clinical status according to MDHAQ scores for physical function, pain and RAPID3. At the same time, most of the problems associated with confounding by indication involve increased adverse events associated with higher doses of a medication in patients with more severe clinical status [58, 59]. In this report, however, few adverse events were seen [42], possibly not more than expected without therapy. Therefore, confounding by indication may not be a prominent problem in the data presented.

A further limitation of observational data in the analysis of results involving a particular therapy (as presented here for prednisone) is that the therapy is not isolated from other therapies while all other variables are kept constant, as in a clinical trial. Therefore, the likelihood that other therapies may affect patient outcomes is substantial. This possibility is documented in the reported series, as the proportion of patients treated with methotrexate was increased from 10% in 1985 to 77% in 2000 (table 6) [66]. These data may explain in large part similar results using low or high doses of prednisone (although other explanations may exist).

Further limitations are seen to the data presented. Since the patients were not randomized, other possible confounding variables, such as age, duration of disease, education level, and other demographic and clinical variables could also affect the results. However, such differences were not seen in comparing patients who were treated with ≥5 versus <5 mg/day of prednisone (data not shown). Another limitation is that adverse events were ascertained by patient self-report, rather than by a systematic review with a health professional, as is performed in a randomized controlled trial protocol. However, the self-report approach appeared valid in another study [71], and patients generally report hypertension, diabetes and cataracts if these conditions develop.

At the same time, it is not feasible to conduct a randomized trial over periods of 3–5 years or longer in a symptomatic disease such as RA, in contrast to asymptomatic individuals who have hypertension or hyperlipidemia. Therefore, long-term observations are required to assess the likelihood of long-term adverse events in RA with any medication, including low-dose glucocorticoids, ideally according to a long-term database of consecutive patients [56]. Although the incidence and prevalence of complications of glucocorticoid therapy were not ascertained systematically as in a randomized trial, bruising and skin-thinning were seen, consistent with other observations of treatment with low-dose prednisone <5 mg/day [74]. The findings are consistent with the comment of Da Silva et al. [73] based on randomized trial data, that 'adverse effects associated with [low-dose prednisone] are modest, and often not statistically different from those of placebo'.

Limitations of Clinical Trials and Advantages of Observational Data

One concern that is often overlooked is that randomized trials also are affected by many limitations [49–55]. Some limitations include patient selection due to exclusion and inclusion criteria, relatively short-term periods of observation when long-term data are needed, reports of patients in groups (as some individuals have better responses in the control group), fixed dosage of medications, limitations on changes in other medications, etc. [49, 50, 52, 75–80].

A database of consecutive patients may provide data that are not available through randomized controlled clinical trials [56], which may be quite relevant to patient care. As noted, a most important consideration involves an attempt to include all consecutive patients – which characterizes the data presented here – to avoid patient selection [56]. Indeed, selection of patients in a traditional clinical case series is a major component of the rationale for a randomized clinical trial, to isolate

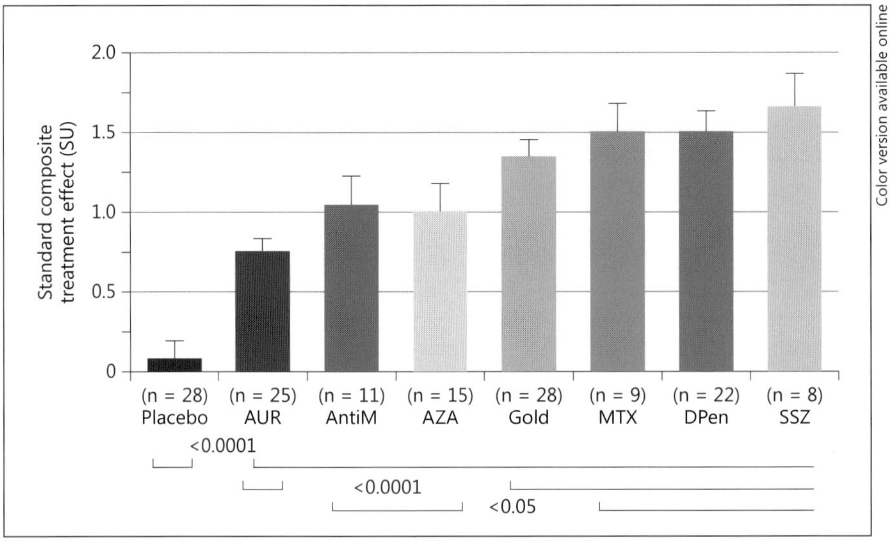

Fig. 4. Comparison of the composite treatment effects of placebo and 7 second-line drugs used to treat RA. Composite treatment effect is the mean of standardized change in tender joint count (adjusted for initial tender joint count, blinding and ESR), ESR and grip strength (adjusted for disease duration and trial length). AUR = Auranofin (oral gold); AntiM = anti-malarials; AZA = azathioprine; MTX = methotrexate; DPen = d-penicillamine; SSZ = sulfasalazine. Source: Felson et al. [81].

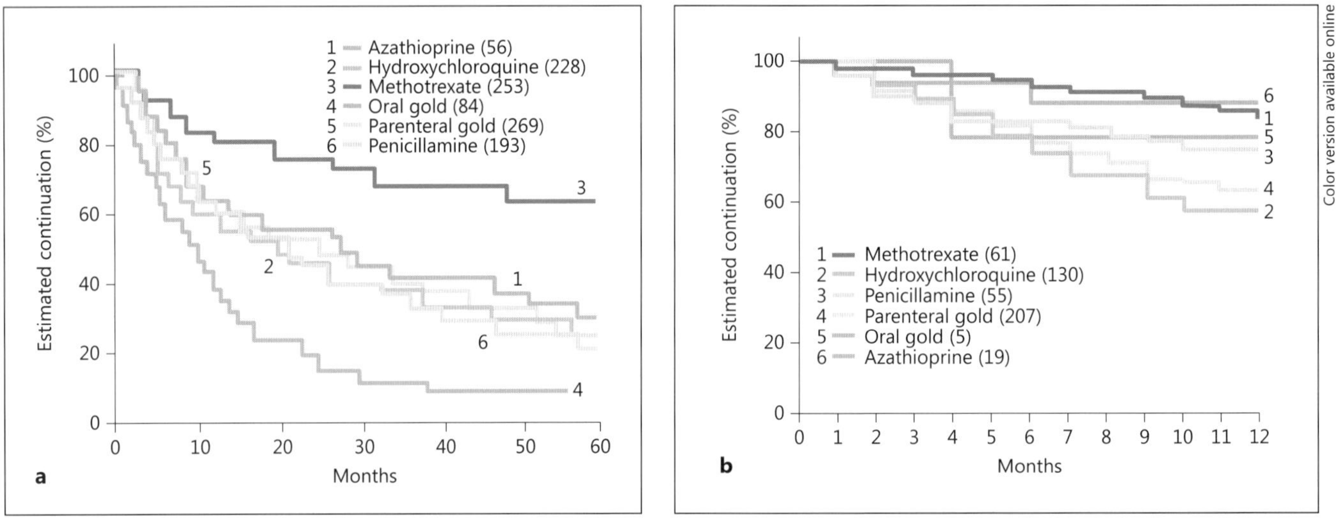

Fig. 5. Probability of continuation of the initial course of the second-line drug in 532 patients with RA over 60 (**a**) and 12 months (**b**). **a** At 60 months, significant differences were seen between methotrexate (top line, most-continued drug) and all other drugs ($p < 0.001$), and between oral gold (bottom line, least-continued drug) and all other drugs ($p < 0.001$); no other differences between drugs were significant. **b** At 12 months, differences between parenteral gold and hydroxychloroquine versus all other drugs were marginally significant ($p = 0.04$); no other significant differences were seen. Source: Pincus et al. [38].

the therapy variable compared to another therapy or a placebo, while all other variables are (hoped to be) similar through randomization [49]. However, observational data may provide considerable information that is not available from clinical trials, particularly if all patients are included.

One example in which observational data have proven more accurate concerning clinical care can be seen in studies of DMARDs in the early 1990s. A meta-analysis of all available randomized trials concerning the efficacy of DMARDs, published in 1990, indicated similar efficacy for methotrexate, injectable gold salts, penicillamine and sulfasalazine [81] (fig. 4). Analyses of a clinical database of 539 patients of 7 rheumatologists reported in 1992 [38] indicated that courses of the initial DMARD over 12 months (1 year) were continued similarly (fig. 5b), consistent with the meta-analysis of all randomized trials [81]. By contrast, analyses of *all* DMARD courses in the identical clinical database patients over 5 years indicated that methotrexate was continued by 50% of patients, compared to fewer than 20% for injectable gold, penicillamine, azathioprine or hydroxychloroquine (fig. 5a) [38], suggesting considerably greater effectiveness of methotrexate. Information regarding therapies over the course of 1 year, whether from clinical trials or clinical practice, does not necessarily accurately depict results over 5 years.

Almost 2 decades later, a 'systematic review' of DMARDs, published in *Annals of Internal Medicine* in 2008, again reported similar efficacy for methotrexate compared to other DMARDs – in this review, sulfasalazine and leflunomide [82]. Again, the conclusions drawn from this systematic review are not consistent with actual care. The proportions of patients taking methotrexate, sulfasalazine and leflunomide, respectively, in the QUEST-RA international database were 83, 43 and 21% in more than 5,000 patients from 15 countries in 2005 [9] (table 1), and 77, 1 and 3% in T.P.'s clinical care in 2000 [66] (table 6), again suggesting that methotrexate is a superior DMARD for most (but not all) patients. Therefore, data from randomized trials – even including meta-analyses and systematic reviews (often regarded as the highest form of evidence [57]) – may give information that is considerably less accurate for clinical practice than data from observational studies [55, 83].

Other limitations of randomized clinical trials are seen. Patient eligibility for a typical RA clinical trial is usually quite restricted. For example, only 5% of patients seen in 2000 in T.P.'s clinic [84] had been eligible for participation in the ATTRACT trial – the first clinical trial to indicate efficacy of a biological agent in RA [85]. Limited numbers of eligible patients is a problem seen in most clinical trials in rheumatic diseases [86].

Another limitation is that clinical trial data are reported for groups of patients, and rarely indicate that more than 80% of individual patients had better outcomes with the preferred treatment for the treatment group, while at least 20% of individual patients in a control group have good responses. For example, in most clinical trials of biological agents in RA, about 60% of patients who take the biological agents experience ACR20 responses, which are seen in about 15% (or more) of patients in the control group [85]. The RA clinical trials which showed greatest efficacy involve a 'treat-to-target' strategy, generally without biological agents – such as FinRACo [87], TICORA [88], BeSt [89], NEO-RACo [100], CAMERA [90] and CIMESTRA [91] – rather than a classical design to compare a biological agent in a fixed dose to a control therapy (which, however, is required to register a new agent). The limited responses in most trials may be explained as much by the presence of joint damage and/or fibromyalgia as by the absence of anti-inflammatory activity [92].

Residual Ongoing Resistance among Physicians to the Use of Low-Dose Methotrexate and Prednisone

The data presented here appear generally to be representative of treatment of RA patients in rheumatology care over the last 3 decades, with increasing use of methotrexate and concomitant low-dose prednisone. Nonetheless, there remains considerable resistance in the medical community to low-dose prednisone and methotrexate, in part for different reasons.

Clinicians recognize the efficacy and effectiveness of prednisone, but most maintain a view of prednisone as a medication with high toxicity, even in low doses. This negative view is often applied to doses of 5 mg/day or less, which are well tolerated over long periods [42], do not affect the hypothalamic-pituitary-adrenal axis [29], and may even be associated with slightly reduced cardiovascular disease [31]. Prednisone remains poorly accepted by the general medical community and even components of the rheumatology community. Even recent EULAR recommendations do not distinguish between the adverse events associated with low-dose versus high-dose glucocorticoids, suggesting that glucocorticoids be avoided or discontinued if possible [7], within 6 months in the most recent version [8]. However, the severe adverse events associated with high-dose prednisone, and even with long-term use of doses such as 10 mg/day, are not seen at 5 mg/day or less (although skin thinning and bruising are not uncommon, particularly in elderly women). Indeed, it may be that 3 mg/day of prednisone is safer than nonsteroidal anti-inflammatory drugs, which are widely prescribed.

Resistance of physicians to methotrexate appears to have a different basis. The efficacy, safety and effectiveness of methotrexate are well established in the medical literature [93]. However, methotrexate continues to be regarded by many physicians as a 'cancer drug', as the primary indications over 30 years involved neoplastic disease.

Analyses of weekly low-dose methotrexate suggest that, at low doses, methotrexate is primarily an anti-inflammatory therapy, with a very different mechanism of action from the cytotoxic effects of high-dose methotrexate to treat neoplastic disease [94, 95]. A reduction in blood counts is not required for effectiveness in RA, and usually is not seen. Indeed, among all patients whose methotrexate was initiated by T.P. between 1990 and 2003, 80% continued methotrexate for longer than 5 years, and no discontinuations were seen because of laboratory abnormalities over 13 years (albeit seeing patients on only 1 day per week) [40]. Very few medications for any chronic disease are continued by 50% of patients for longer than 5 years. Weekly low-dose methotrexate (as well as 3 mg/day of prednisone) would appear as safe as or safer than most, if not all, antibiotics, as well as most, if not all, non-steroidal anti-inflammatory drugs, antihypertensive or antidepressant medications [80].

It has been suggested that an 'n-of-1 trial' of low-dose prednisone and/or methotrexate might be a reasonable, cost-effective alternative to expensive tests to establish a definitive diagnosis of RA for an individual patient [96]. Historically, it was very important to establish a relatively certain diagnosis of RA, in the absence of a 'gold standard' diagnostic marker, as the traditional primary DMARDs from the 1960s to the 1980s, parenteral gold therapy and penicillamine, were considerably less safe therapies than low-dose methotrexate or prednisone. Many rheumatologists cared for patients who developed glomerulonephritis or aplastic anemia associated with gold or penicillamine therapies, often without warning or any hint of toxicity, until acute severe illness and death resulted.

Acute toxicity is not seen with weekly low-dose methotrexate or daily low-dose prednisone. Of course, adverse events and toxicities are seen, but it may be defensible or even desirable simply to treat patients who might have inflammatory arthritis with an 'n-of-1' trial, monitoring patients quantitatively through joint counts, laboratory tests, and/or a simple self-report questionnaire, such as MDHAQ/RAPID3. Laboratory tests are not as informative as in earlier decades: most RA patients seen in the1950s had elevated ESR and/or CRP, but only about half have elevated acute-phase reactants today [97, 98].

Concluding Thoughts

It is important to recognize that the phenomena of the reduction of prednisone dosage along with the increasing use of methotrexate could not be documented in clinical trials, but only with long-term observational data. Clinical trials are essential to establish initially the efficacy and safety of a therapy. Furthermore, it might have been possible, as the data were evolving clinically, to have performed, say, in 1990 a clinical trial of, say, 3 versus 5 versus 10 mg/day of prednisone concomitant with methotrexate therapy. However, resources for such a clinical trial were not available.

It is not too late for such a clinical trial, as some rheumatologists may continue to treat RA patients with far higher prednisone doses than may be needed, with a greater likelihood of adverse events. For example, 30 mg/day of prednisone, while generally safe over a period of 1 or 2 weeks, may be associated with adverse events such as uncontrolled hunger and even psychotic episodes in some patients. Such episodes could be avoided by never using these doses except in patients with extreme life-threatening disease, but results of the 'COBRA-light' trial might support initial use of these doses as more efficacious than an initial 3 mg dose [99]. Further studies appear indicated.

This review indicates that long-term, low-dose prednisone, at doses of <5 mg/day, appears feasible and effective for many patients with RA, including an initial dose of 3 mg/day. Indefinite continuation is possible in many if not most patients, particularly with concomitant methotrexate, another DMARD or biological agent. Improvements in methodologies of both observational studies and clinical trials, and further clinical research using both of these methodologies, will advance knowledge concerning long-term use of <5 mg/day of prednisone, toward better patient care and outcomes. Nonetheless, it may never be possible to isolate prednisone (or methotrexate or a biological agent or physical therapy or any single variable) for the treatment of RA (or any chronic disease) over 5 years or longer, as logistic, medical and ethical considerations would require that multiple therapies be used for patient care. These limitations should not deter efforts to characterize better the most effective strategies using observational data to achieve optimal patient outcomes in RA.

References

1 Hench PS, Kendall EC, Slocumb CH, Polley HF: The effect of a hormone of the adrenal cortex (17-hydroxy-11-dehydrocorticosterone; compound E) and of the pituitary adrenocorticotropic hormone on rheumatoid arthritis. Proc Staff Meet Mayo Clin 1949;24:181.

2 Hench PS: The reversibility of certain rheumatic and non-rheumatic conditions by the use of cortisone or of the pituitary adrenocorticotropic hormone. Ann Intern Med 1952;36:1–38.

3 Joint Committee of the Medical Research Council and Nuffield Foundation: A comparison of cortisone and aspirin in the treatment of early cases of rheumatoid arthritis. Br Med J 1954;29:1223–1227.
4 Polley HF, Slocumb CH, Ward LE, Hench PS: Recognition and treatment of patients with chronic hypercortisonism. Ann Rheum Dis 1955;14:416–417.
5 de Andrade JR, McCormick JN, Hill AGS: Small doses of prednisolone in the management of rheumatoid arthritis. Ann Rheum Dis 1964;23:158–162.
6 Benedek TG: History of the development of corticosteroid therapy. Clin Exp Rheumatol 2011;29(5 suppl 68):5–12.
7 Gorter SL, Bijlsma JW, Cutolo M, Gomez-Reino J, Kouloumas M, Smolen JS, et al: Current evidence for the management of rheumatoid arthritis with glucocorticoids: a systematic literature review informing the EULAR recommendations for the management of rheumatoid arthritis. Ann Rheum Dis 2010;69:1010–1014.
8 Smolen JS, Landewe R, Breedveld FC, Buch M, Burmester G, Dougados M, et al: EULAR recommendations for the management of rheumatoid arthritis with synthetic and biological disease-modifying antirheumatic drugs: 2013 update. Ann Rheum Dis 2014;73:492–509.
9 Sokka T, Kautiainen H, Toloza S, Makinen H, Verstappen SMM, Hetland ML, et al: QUEST-RA: quantitative clinical assessment of patients with rheumatoid arthritis seen in standard rheumatology care in 15 countries. Ann Rheum Dis 2007;66:1491–1496.
10 Sokka T, Toloza S, Cutolo M, Kautiainen H, Makinen H, Gogus F, et al: Women, men, and rheumatoid arthritis: analyses of disease activity, disease characteristics, and treatments in the QUEST-RA Study. Arthritis Res Ther 2009;11:R7.
11 Harris ED Jr, Emkey RD, Nichols JE, Newberg A: Low dose prednisone therapy in rheumatoid arthritis: a double blind study. J Rheumatol 1983;10:713–721.
12 Yelin E, Meenan R, Nevitt M, Epstein W: Work disability in rheumatoid arthritis: effects of disease, social, and work factors. Ann Intern Med 1980;93:551–556.
13 Pincus T, Callahan LF, Sale WG, Brooks AL, Payne LE, Vaughn WK: Severe functional declines, work disability, and increased mortality in seventy-five rheumatoid arthritis patients studied over nine years. Arthritis Rheum 1984;27:864–872.
14 Scott DL, Grindulis KA, Struthers GR, Coulton BL, Popert AJ, Bacon PA: Progression of radiological changes in rheumatoid arthritis. Ann Rheum Dis 1984;43:8–17.
15 Kirwan JR: The effects of glucocorticoids on joint destruction in rheumatoid arthritis. N Engl J Med 1995;333:142–146.
16 Boers M, Verhoeven AC, Markusse HM, van de Laar MAFJ, Westhovens R, van Denderen JC, et al: Randomised comparison of combined step-down prednisolone, methotrexate and sulphasalazine with sulphasalazine alone in early rheumatoid arthritis. Lancet 1997;350:309–318.
17 van Everdingen AA, Jacobs JWG, van Reesema DRS, Bijlsma JWJ: Low-dose prednisone therapy for patients with early active rheumatoid arthritis: clinical efficacy, disease-modifying properties, and side effects. Ann Intern Med 2002;136:1–12.
18 Svensson B, Boonen A, Albertsson K, van der Heijde D, Keller C, Hafstrom I: Low-dose prednisolone in addition to the initial disease-modifying antirheumatic drug in patients with early active rheumatoid arthritis reduces joint destruction and increases the remission rate: a two-year randomized trial. Arthritis Rheum 2005;52:3360–3370.
19 Wassenberg S, Rau R, Steinfeld P, Zeidler H: Very low-dose prednisolone in early rheumatoid arthritis retards radiographic progression over two years: a multicenter, double-blind, placebo-controlled trial. Arthritis Rheum 2005;52:3371–3380.
20 Buttgereit F, Doering G, Schaeffler A, Witte S, Sierakowski S, Gromnica-Ihle E, et al: Efficacy of modified-release versus standard prednisone to reduce duration of morning stiffness of the joints in rheumatoid arthritis (CAPRA-1): a double-blind, randomised controlled trial. Lancet 2008;371:205–214.
21 Pincus T, Swearingen CJ, Luta G, Sokka T: Efficacy of prednisone 1–4 mg/day in patients with rheumatoid arthritis: a randomised, double-blind, placebo controlled withdrawal clinical trial. Ann Rheum Dis 2009;68:1715–1720.
22 Montecucco C, Todoerti M, Sakellariou G, Scire CA, Caporali R: Low-dose oral prednisone improves clinical and ultrasonographic remission rates in early rheumatoid arthritis: results of a 12-month open-label randomised study. Arthritis Res Ther 2012;14:R112.
23 Bakker MF, Jacobs JW, Welsing PM, Verstappen SM, Tekstra J, Ton E, et al: Low-dose prednisone inclusion in a methotrexate-based, tight control strategy for early rheumatoid arthritis: a randomized trial. Ann Intern Med 2012;156:329–339.
24 Buttgereit F, Mehta D, Kirwan J, Szechinski J, Boers M, Alten RE, et al: Low-dose prednisone chronotherapy for rheumatoid arthritis: a randomised clinical trial (CAPRA-2). Ann Rheum Dis 2013;72:204–210.
25 Kirwan JR, Bijlsma JW, Boers M, Shea BJ: Effects of glucocorticoids on radiological progression in rheumatoid arthritis. Cochrane Database Syst Rev 2007:CD006356.
26 Danowski TS, Bonessi JV, Sabeh G, Sutton RD, Webster MW Jr, Sarver ME: Probabilities of pituitary-adrenal responsiveness after steroid therapy. Ann Intern Med 1964;61:11–26.
27 Wood JB, Frankland AW, James VH, Landon J: A rapid test of adrenocortical function. Lancet 1965;1:243–245.
28 Daly JR, Myles AB, Bacon PA, Beardwell CG, Savage O: Pituitary adrenal function during corticosteroid withdrawal in rheumatoid arthritis. Ann Rheum Dis 1967;26:18–25.
29 LaRochelle GE Jr, LaRochelle AG, Ratner RE, Borenstein DG: Recovery of the hypothalamic-pituitary-adrenal (HPA) axis in patients with rheumatic diseases receiving low-dose prednisone. Am J Med 1993;95:258–264.
30 Saag KG, Koehnke R, Caldwell JR, Brasington R, Burmeister LF, Zimmerman B, et al: Low dose long-term corticosteroid therapy in rheumatoid arthritis: an analysis of serious adverse events. Am J Med 1994;96:115–123.
31 Wei L, MacDonald TM, Walker BR: Taking glucocorticoids by prescription is associated with subsequent cardiovascular disease. Ann Intern Med 2004;141:764–770.
32 Laan RF, van Riel PL, van de Putte LB, van Erning LJ, van't Hof MA, Lemmens JA: Low-dose prednisone induces rapid reversible axial bone loss in patients with rheumatoid arthritis: a randomized, controlled study. Ann Intern Med 1993;119:963–968.
33 Pincus T, Brooks RH, Callahan LF: Prediction of long-term mortality in patients with rheumatoid arthritis according to simple questionnaire and joint count measures. Ann Intern Med 1994;120:26–34.
34 Wolfe F, Mitchell DM, Sibley JT, Fries JF, Bloch DA, Williams CA, et al: The mortality of rheumatoid arthritis. Arthritis Rheum 1994;37:481–494.
35 Hoffmeister RT: Methotrexate therapy in rheumatoid arthritis: 15 years experience. Am J Med 1983;75(suppl 6A):69–73.
36 Hoffmeister RT: Methotrexate in rheumatoid arthritis (abstract). Arthritis Rheum 1972;15(suppl):S114.
37 Weinblatt ME, Coblyn JS, Fox DA, Fraser PA, Holdsworth DE, Glass DN, et al: Efficacy of low-dose methotrexate in rheumatoid arthritis. N Engl J Med 1985;312:818–822.
38 Pincus T, Marcum SB, Callahan LF: Long-term drug therapy for rheumatoid arthritis in seven rheumatology private practices. II. Second-line drugs and prednisone. J Rheumatol 1992;19:1885–1894.
39 Pincus T, Gibson KA, Castrejón I: Update on methotrexate as the anchor drug for rheumatoid arthritis. Bull Hosp Jt Dis 2013;71(suppl 1):S9–S19.
40 Yazici Y, Sokka T, Kautiainen H, Swearingen C, Kulman I, Pincus T: Long term safety of methotrexate in routine clinical care: discontinuation is unusual and rarely the result of laboratory abnormalities. Ann Rheum Dis 2005;64:207–211.
41 Pincus T, Castrejon I, Sokka T: Long-term prednisone in doses of less than 5 mg/day for treatment of rheumatoid arthritis: personal experience over 25 years. Clin Exp Rheumatol 2011;29(5 suppl 68):S130–S138.
42 Pincus T, Sokka T, Castrejón I, Cutolo M: Decline of mean initial prednisone dosage from 10.3 to 3.6 mg/day to treat rheumatoid arthritis between 1980 and 2004 in one clinical setting, with long-term effectiveness of dosages less than 5 mg/day. Arthritis Care Res 2013;65:729–736.

43 Sokka T, Pincus T: Ascendancy of weekly low-dose methotrexate in usual care of rheumatoid arthritis from 1980 to 2004 at two sites in Finland and the United States. Rheumatology (Oxford) 2008;47:1543–1547.
44 Pincus T, Swearingen CJ: The HAQ compared with the MDHAQ: 'keep it simple, stupid' (KISS), with feasibility and clinical value as primary criteria for patient questionnaires in usual clinical care. Rheum Dis Clin North Am 2009;35:787–798.
45 Pincus T, Swearingen C, Wolfe F: Toward a multidimensional health assessment questionnaire (MDHAQ): assessment of advanced activities of daily living and psychological status in the patient friendly health assessment questionnaire format. Arthritis Rheum 1999; 42:2220–2230.
46 Pincus T, Sokka T, Kautiainen H: Further development of a physical function scale on a multidimensional health assessment questionnaire for standard care of patients with rheumatic diseases. J Rheumatol 2005;32: 1432–1439.
47 Pincus T, Yazici Y, Bergman MJ: RAPID3, an index to assess and monitor patients with rheumatoid arthritis, without formal joint counts: similar results to DAS28 and CDAI in clinical trials and clinical care. Rheum Dis Clin North Am 2009;35:773–778.
48 Sackett DL, Rosenberg WM, Gray JM, Haynes RB, Richardson WS: Evidence based medicine: what it is and what it isn't: it's about integrating individual clinical expertise and the best external evidence. Br Med J 1996;312: 71–72.
49 Feinstein AR: An additional basic science for clinical medicine. II. The limitations of randomized trials. Ann Intern Med 1983;99:544–550.
50 Pincus T: Limitations of randomized controlled clinical trials to recognize possible advantages of combination therapies in rheumatic diseases. Semin Arthritis Rheum 1993; 23(suppl 1):2–10.
51 Pincus T, Callahan LF: Prognostic markers of activity and damage in rheumatoid arthritis: why clinical trials and inception cohort studies indicate more favorable outcomes than studies of patients with established disease. Br J Rheumatol 1995;34:196–199.
52 Pincus T, Stein CM: Why randomized controlled clinical trials do not depict accurately long-term outcomes in rheumatoid arthritis: some explanations and suggestions for future studies. Clin Exp Rheumatol 1997;15(suppl 17):S27–S38.
53 Kaptchuk TJ: The double-blind, randomized, placebo-controlled trial: gold standard or golden calf? J Clin Epidemiol 2001;54:541–549.
54 Pincus T, Sokka T: Should contemporary rheumatoid arthritis clinical trials be more like standard patient care and vice versa? Ann Rheum Dis 2004;63(suppl II):ii32–ii39.
55 Pincus T, Sokka T: Clinical trials in rheumatic diseases: designs and limitations. Rheum Dis Clin North Am 2004;30:701–704.
56 Moses LE: The series of consecutive cases as a device for assessing outcomes of intervention. N Engl J Med 1984;311:705–710.
57 Lau J, Ioannidis JP, Schmid CH: Summing up evidence: one answer is not always enough. Lancet 1998;351:123–127.
58 Psaty BM, Koepsell TD, Lin D, Weiss NS, Siscovick DS, Rosendaal FR, et al: Assessment and control for confounding by indication in observational studies. J Am Geriatr Soc 1999; 47:749–754.
59 Landewe RB: The benefits of early treatment in rheumatoid arthritis: confounding by indication, and the issue of timing. Arthritis Rheum 2003;48:1–5.
60 OCEBM Levels of Evidence Working Group: The Oxford 2011 Levels of Evidence. Oxford, Centre for Evidence-Based Medicine, 2011. http://www.cebm.net/index.aspx?o=5653.
61 Howick J: The Philosophy of Evidence-Based Medicine. Oxford, Wiley-Blackwell, 2011.
62 Smith GCS, Pell JP: Parachute use to prevent death and major trauma related to gravitational challenge: systematic review of randomised controlled trials. BMJ 2003;327: 1459–1461.
63 Glasziou P, Chalmers I, Rawlins M, McCulloch P: When are randomised trials unnecessary? Picking signal from noise. BMJ 2007; 334:349–351.
64 Aronson JK, Hauben M: Anecdotes that provide definitive evidence. BMJ 2006;333:1267–1269.
65 Wolfe F, Hawley DJ: Remission in rheumatoid arthritis. J Rheumatol 1985;12:245–252.
66 Pincus T, Sokka T, Kautiainen H: Patients seen for standard rheumatoid arthritis care have significantly better articular, radiographic, laboratory, and functional status in 2000 than in 1985. Arthritis Rheum 2005;52: 1009–1019.
67 Pincus T, Stein CM, Wolfe F: 'No evidence of disease' in rheumatoid arthritis using methotrexate in combination with other drugs: a contemporary goal for rheumatology care? Clin Exp Rheumatol 1997;15:591–596.
68 Pincus T, Sokka T, Stein CM: Are long-term very low doses of prednisone for patients with rheumatoid arthritis as helpful as high doses are harmful? Ann Intern Med 2002;136:76–78.
69 Silman A, Davies P, Currey HLF, Evans SJW: Is rheumatoid arthritis becoming less severe? J Chronic Dis 1983;36:891–897.
70 Spector TD, Hart DJ, Powell RJ: Prevalence of rheumatoid arthritis and rheumatoid factor in women: evidence for a secular decline. Ann Rheum Dis 1993;52:254–257.
71 Porter DR, Capell HA, McInnes I, Munro R, Madhok R, Hunter JA et al: Is rheumatoid arthritis becoming a milder disease? Or are we starting second-line therapy in patients with milder disease? Br J Rheumatol 1996;35: 1305–1308.
72 Welsing PMJ, Fransen J, van Riel PLCM: Is the disease course of rheumatoid arthritis becoming milder? Time trends since 1985 in an inception cohort of early rheumatoid arthritis. Arthritis Rheum 2005;52:2616–2624.
73 Da Silva JA, Jacobs JW, Kirwan JR, Boers M, Saag KG, Ines LB, et al: Safety of low dose glucocorticoid treatment in rheumatoid arthritis: published evidence and prospective trial data. Ann Rheum Dis 2006;65:285–293.
74 Huscher D, Thiele K, Gromnica-Ihle E, Hein G, Demary W, Dreher R, et al: Dose-related patterns of glucocorticoid-induced side effects. Ann Rheum Dis 2009;68:1119–1124.
75 Pincus T: Rheumatoid arthritis: disappointing long-term outcomes despite successful short-term clinical trials. J Clin Epidemiol 1988;41:1037–1041.
76 Fleming TR, DeMets DL: Surrogate end points in clinical trials: are we being misled? Ann Intern Med 1996;125:605–613.
77 Pincus T: Limitations of randomized clinical trials in chronic diseases: explanations and recommendations. Adv Mind Body Med 2002;18:14–21.
78 Fransen J, van Riel PLCM: Are better endpoints and better design of clinical trials needed? Best Pract Res Clin Rheumatol 2004;18: 97–109.
79 Pincus T, Yazici Y, Sokka T: Are excellent systematic reviews of clinical trials useful for patient care? Nat Clin Pract Rheumatol 2008;4: 294–295.
80 Pincus T, Furer V, Sokka T: Underestimation of the efficacy, effectiveness, tolerability, and safety of weekly low-dose methotrexate in information presented to physicians and patients. Clin Exp Rheumatol 2010;28(5 suppl 61):S68–S79.
81 Felson DT, Anderson JJ, Meenan RF: The comparative efficacy and toxicity of second-line drugs in rheumatoid arthritis: results of two metaanalyses. Arthritis Rheum 1990;33: 1449–1461.
82 Donahue KE, Gartlehner G, Jonas DE, Lux LJ, Thieda P, Jonas BL, et al: Systematic review: comparative effectiveness and harms of disease-modifying medications for rheumatoid arthritis. Ann Intern Med 2008;148:124–134.
83 Pincus T: Limitations to standard randomized controlled clinical trials to evaluate combination therapies in rheumatic diseases. Agents Actions Suppl 1993;44:83–91.
84 Sokka T, Pincus T: Eligibility of patients in routine care for major clinical trials of anti-tumor necrosis factor alpha agents in rheumatoid arthritis. Arthritis Rheum 2003;48:313–318.
85 Maini R, St Clair EW, Breedveld F, Furst D, Kalden J, Weisman M, et al: Infliximab (chimeric anti-tumour necrosis factor alpha monoclonal antibody) versus placebo in rheumatoid arthritis patients receiving concomitant methotrexate: a randomized phase III trial. Lancet 1999;354:1932–1939.
86 Sokka T, Pincus T: Most patients receiving routine care for rheumatoid arthritis in 2001 did not meet inclusion criteria for most recent clinical trials or American College of Rheumatology criteria for remission. J Rheumatol 2003;30:1138–1146.

87 Möttönen T, Hannonen P, Leirisalo-Repo M, Nissilä M, Kautiainen H, Korpela M, et al: Comparison of combination therapy with single-drug therapy in early rheumatoid arthritis: a randomised trial. FIN-RACo trial group. Lancet 1999;353:1568–1573.
88 Grigor C, Capell H, Stirling A, McMahon AD, Lock P, Vallance R, et al: Effect of a treatment strategy of tight control for rheumatoid arthritis (the TICORA study): a single-blind randomised controlled trial. Lancet 2004;364: 263–269.
89 Goekoop-Ruiterman YPM, de Vries-Bouwstra JK, Allaart CF, van Zeben D, Kerstens PJSM, Hazes JMW, et al: Clinical and radiographic outcomes of four different treatment strategies in patients with early rheumatoid arthritis (the BeSt study): a randomized, controlled trial. Arthritis Rheum 2005;52:3381–3390.
90 Verstappen SMM, Jacobs JWG, van der Veen MJ, Heurkens AHM, Schenk Y, ter Borg EJ, et al: Intensive treatment with methotrexate in early rheumatoid arthritis: aiming for remission – Computer Assisted Management in Early Rheumatoid Arthritis (CAMERA, an open-label strategy trial). Ann Rheum Dis 2007;66:1443–1449.
91 Hetland ML, Stengaard-Pedersen K, Junker P, Lottenburger T, Hansen I, Andersen LS, et al: Aggressive combination therapy with intra-articular glucocorticoid injections and conventional disease-modifying anti-rheumatic drugs in early rheumatoid arthritis: second-year clinical and radiographic results from the CIMESTRA study. Ann Rheum Dis 2008;67:815–822.
92 Tymms K, Zochling J, Scott J, Bird P, Burnet S, de JJ, et al: Barriers to optimal disease control for rheumatoid arthritis patients with moderate and high disease activity. Arthritis Care Res (Hoboken) 2014;66:190–196.
93 Braun J, Pincus T, Cronstein B: Methotrexate in rheumatic diseases. Clin Exp Rheumatol 2010;28(5 suppl 61).
94 Cronstein BN: Molecular therapeutics: methotrexate and its mechanism of action. Arthritis Rheum 1996;39:1951–1960.
95 Chan ESL, Cronstein BN: Molecular action of methotrexate in inflammatory diseases. Arthritis Res 2002;4:266–273.
96 Pincus T, Huizinga TWJ, Yazici Y: N-of-1 trial of low-dose methotrexate and/or prednisolone in lieu of anti-CCP, MRI, or ultrasound, as first option in suspected rheumatoid arthritis? J Rheumatol 2007;34:250–252.
97 Sokka T, Pincus T: Erythrocyte sedimentation rate, C-reactive protein, or rheumatoid factor are normal at presentation in 35%–45% of patients with rheumatoid arthritis seen between 1980 and 2004: analyses from Finland and the United States. J Rheumatol 2009;36:1387–1390.
98 Abelson B, Sokka T, Pincus T: Declines in erythrocyte sedimentation rates in patients with rheumatoid arthritis over the second half of the 20th century. J Rheumatol 2009; 36:1596–1599.
99 den Uyl D, Ter Wee M, Boers M, Kerstens P, Voskuyl A, Nurmohamed M, et al: A non-inferiority trial of an attenuated combination strategy ('COBRA-light') compared to the original COBRA strategy: clinical results after 26 weeks. Ann Rheum Dis 2014;73: 1071–1078.
100 Leirisalo-Repo M, et al: Infliximab for 6 months added on combination therapy in early rheumatoid arthritis: 2-year results from an investigator-initiated, randomised, double-blind, placebo-controlled study (the NEO-RACo Study). Ann Rheum Dis 2013;72:851–857.

Observational Studies and Clinical Experience with Low-Dose Glucocorticoids

NeuroImmunoModulation

Neuroimmunomodulation 2015;22:104–111
DOI: 10.1159/000362730

Published online: September 12, 2014

Oral Low-Dose Glucocorticoids Should Be Included in Any Recommendation for the Use of Non-Biologic and Biologic Disease-Modifying Antirheumatic Drugs in the Treatment of Rheumatoid Arthritis

Roberto Caporali[a] Monica Todoerti[a] Carlo Alberto Scirè[a]
Carlomaurizio Montecucco[a] Maurizio Cutolo[b]

[a]Division of Rheumatology, University of Pavia, IRCCS Policlinico San Matteo Foundation, Pavia, and
[b]Research Laboratory and Division of Clinical Rheumatology, Department of Internal Medicine, University of Genoa, Genoa, Italy

Key Words
Glucocorticoids · Disease-modifying antirheumatic drugs · Rheumatoid arthritis

Abstract
At present, growing scientific evidence from the medical literature and expert opinion provides strong consideration for a mandatory role of glucocorticoids (GCs) in the management of rheumatoid arthritis (RA). Earlier application strategies were based on initial high doses, with subsequent tapering schedules, resulting in dose-related side effects. Recent low-dose GC schemes are more feasible in routine care, while providing evidence of clinical, functional and structural efficacy. Thus, initial low-dose GC 'bridging' treatment on a disease-modifying antirheumatic drug background should be included in any existing recommendations for RA management, as very recently advocated by the EULAR Task Force 2013 updated guidelines. Long-term low-dose therapy appears to provide acceptable safety, leading to long-standing slowing of structural damage, seen even after GC therapy withdrawal. Gaps in knowledge about the optimal method to taper and possibly discontinue GC treatment remain, and this topic should be addressed in clinical trials and observational studies. Recent efforts in GC medication have also included the introduction of a modified-release drug formulation capable of drug delivery consistent with chronobiological pathogenetic rhythms of disease, which has been quite efficacious in controlling the signs and symptoms related to pathways of circadian cytokines. Long-term data will further clarify the add-on benefits of such modified-release formulations.

Introduction

At present the management of patients with rheumatoid arthritis (RA) is based on early methotrexate (MTX) and other disease-modifying antirheumatic drugs (DMARDs), and biological agents in incomplete responders, supported by recommendations of national and multinational organizations [1–3]. Recently published classification criteria allow early recognition and early treatment of RA patients [4, 5]. Clinical practice is based on both systematic literature research and expert opinion,

KARGER

E-Mail karger@karger.com
www.karger.com/nim

1021–7401/14/0222–0104$39.50/0

Roberto Caporali, MD
Division of Rheumatology, IRCCS Policlinico S. Matteo
P. le Golgi 2
IT–27100 Pavia (Italy)
E-Mail caporali@smatteo.pv.it

thus combining the best of objective knowledge in the field with the expertise of specialists [1–3]. A favorable effectiveness profile of such DMARDs has been demonstrated: well-recognized clinical, sub-clinical and structural effects are accompanied by relatively acceptable safety profiles, so that these agents represent the mainstay of RA treatment. Along with this evidence, re-analysis of past and new emerging data concerning the efficacy of traditional agents such as glucocorticoids (GCs) has prompted re-examination and re-evaluation of GCs in association with DMARDs in the management of RA.

GC Use in the Existing Guidelines

A EULAR task force has developed evidence-based recommendations for the best use and management of GC therapy in all rheumatic diseases [6], and subsequent guidelines focused on GC use in RA patients [7]. The combination of systematically retrieved research evidence and expert opinion consensus were the leading principles of both sets of recommendations [6, 7]. In addition, the recently published 2013 update of EULAR recommendations for RA management addressed GC treatment as a separate topic, due to the proven clinical, functional and structural efficacy of GCs when combined with DMARDs [8]. These recommendations state that low-dose GC 'should be considered as part of the initial treatment strategy', rather than 'providing benefit', as stated in the previous version [9]. The time frame of the 'short-term period of initial GC therapy' was specifically defined as lasting 'up to 6 months', suggesting tapering as soon as is clinically possible.

In contrast to the European prospective, the American College of Rheumatology (ACR) guidelines for RA treatment and their recent 2012 update continued not to address the role of GCs [10, 11]. The original 2008 ACR guidelines explicitly stated that GCs, 'despite their frequent use in RA, were not part of the ACR charge and were not included in these recommendations' [10]. The 2012 ACR update states that 'the use of other anti-inflammatory medications, such as non-steroidal anti-inflammatory drugs and intra-articular and oral GCs, were not within the purview of the update, although these may be important components of RA treatment and could also be included in separate reviews or recommendations' [11].

Other guidelines have been produced, too. The National Institute for Clinical Excellence (NICE) in the UK advises combination therapy with GCs in different ways in different clinical circumstances, such as early versus established disease and short versus long-term GC medication [12]. Translating evidence into recommendations, they consider treatment with GCs via oral, intramuscular or intra-articular routes, to improve symptoms rapidly in people with newly diagnosed RA, if they are not already receiving GCs as part of DMARD combination therapy. Short-term GC treatment could be considered even for managing flares in people with both recent-onset or established disease, to decrease inflammation rapidly. In people with established RA, continued long-term treatment with GCs would be acceptable only if long-term complications have been fully discussed and all other treatment options, including biological agents, have been offered.

Thus, European recommendations – particularly the recent 2013 EULAR update and UK guidelines – note the value of GC co-medication in the management of RA, based on studies which showed that adding GCs to DMARDs is quite beneficial to better disease outcomes. Additional comprehensive information is found in a very recent systematic literature review by Gaujoux-Viala et al. [13], supporting GCs as add-on therapy on a DMARD background, whilst GC monotherapy is generally not advised [14].

Literature Evidence Concerning GCs in RA over Long Periods

Since their first use in the mid-1950s, conflicting opinions have been held about GC medication because of the potential side effects of long-term use and higher dosages. In the controlled setting of clinical trials, selected patients have benefited from different GC schedules, including both initially high/rapidly tapered regimens and chronic lower dosages, suggesting that both strategies have an acceptable risk/benefit profile and disease-modifying properties [15]. In actual practice, aggressive high-dose GC management is not appropriate, and attention has shifted to low-dose GC strategies, for which available literature supports acceptable safety [16, 17]. Thus, in everyday clinical practice, a clear trend in reduced GC dose has gradually appeared over the last decades; concomitantly, conventional and then biological DMARD agents have been incorporated into routine management of inflammatory rheumatic diseases with a relevant increase over time in the proportion of patients taking them. This might explain in part the gradual reduction of the prednisone dose over this period, along with more favorable outcomes and better patient status in recent years [18]. The available data document that prednisone at doses <5 mg/day over long periods appears acceptable and effective for many real-life patients with RA at present [19], as confirmed in the more up-to-date reference of the 25-year experience of one rheumatologist [17]. Rapid step-down strategies, as adopted in COBRA and COBRA-like regimens (BeSt trial), are based on an initial aggressive therapeutic approach in patients with poor prognostic factors [20, 21]. In the BeSt trial, patients initially treated with aggressive combination therapy strategies (i.e. DMARD in combination with a biologic agent or with an initial high GC dose) exhibited more rapid functional improvement, with significantly better results for up to 1 year of follow-up as compared to other treatment schedules of DMARDs in sequence or in combinations from the beginning, although all groups were similar after 2 years. Combination therapy with high-dose GCs provided similar short-term and long-term results as combination treatment initially with infliximab. A meta-analysis showed that add-on GC therapy could be as effective as DMARD combination therapy (plus other synthetic DMARDs or plus biologic agents) in preventing structural progression [22]. In actual practice, some patients may have co-morbidities that involve absolute or relative contraindications to a high GC dose. Therefore, other treatment regimens focused on lower GC dosages were recently explored in the management of RA patients. An attenuated COBRA regimen ('COBRA-light strategy') using lower prednisolone doses, starting at 30 mg/day and tapered to 7.5 mg/day in 9 weeks, plus MTX escalated to 25 mg/week in 9 weeks, has recently been published, showing non-inferiority to the original COBRA schedule in terms of clinical remission achievement. This could be the starting point to further assess lighter GC protocols [23] (see the article by Rasch et al. in this volume). The first randomized controlled trial (RCT) by Kirwan et al. [24] in 1995 indicated that combination therapy with DMARDs and low-dose oral prednisolone could reduce and prevent structural progression. Several subsequent reports confirm these results [25–27]. All published RCTs confirm the more rapid achievement of better results in patients treated with low-dose GC combination therapy in clinical, functional and structural endpoints. Lower benefit is seen in cases of long-standing disease, indicating that the principle of the 'window of opportunity' pertains to GC medication: the earlier, the better [28, 29]. The structural effects of GCs are more evident when administered in the early phase of the disease. Protocols aiming at pre-defined targets, i.e. within a tight control and treat-to-target management strategy, provide optimal results. In the CAMERA-II clinical trial, adding prednisone at a dosage of 10 mg/day significantly increased MTX effectiveness: erosive joint damage after 2 years, the primary outcome, together with disease activity and functional disability were significantly lower with MTX and prednisone versus MTX and placebo [30]. In addition, a recent trial by our group indicated greater efficacy of GC co-medication over MTX monotherapy in reducing the signs of active synovitis indicated by a power Doppler signal, which is a well-recognized predictive factor for future structural damage and clinical relapse during disease remission phases [31–34]. The combined clinical and ultrasound outcome was more than double in the MTX + low-dose prednisone group than in the MTX monotherapy group. The efficacy of GCs is also supported by a meta-analysis where pooled data have been adjusted for heterogeneity of designs and populations [35]. Fifteen trials have been involved for a total of 1,414 RA patients, considering all trials where either low-dose oral steroids (<10 mg prednisone equivalent) or initial high-dose tapered schedules, as monotherapy or in combination with DMARDs, were compared to placebo or active treatments. GC co-therapy, regardless of the selected dose between 5 and 10 mg/day, was associated with a significant reduction of radiographic progression (which was chosen as the primary outcome in most studies) both in the first and second year of follow-up. Such results refer primarily to patients with early-onset RA, with a mean symptom duration of less than 2 years. The only two studies that enrolled patients with established disease (more than 2 years of disease duration) did not show similar positive findings, although confounding factors other than GC therapy also should be considered [28, 29]. The authors concluded that in early RA patients, low-dose oral GCs reduce radiographic progression over up to 2 years of follow-up. Further, long-term follow-up studies evaluating the effects of treatment strategies that include GCs, either at low or higher dosages, given early in the course of disease, indicate a slowing of radiographic joint damage even after the end of the study protocol [36–39]. Thus, it appears that slowing joint damage persists, even after GC therapy has been stopped – a true disease-modifying effect that has not been shown with other DMARD therapies [40]. In this regard, indications to stop or not and strategies to taper GCs might vary, but are currently mostly described based on expert opinion [17, 41, 42]. A recent systematic literature review addressed the influence of tapering regimens on successful GC withdrawal, as well as clinical outcomes [41]. Despite a thorough and careful systematic literature review, data for tapering GCs in RA were heterogeneous and incomplete, so that there is presently no evidence-based answer to the question. However, it may not be necessary to taper below 3 mg/day [18].

Management of GC withdrawal could be more difficult when specifically considering patients under biologic treatment. At present, several trials have investigated the possibility of tapering and stopping biological agents when disease control has been successfully achieved. Most of these studies allowed concomitant GC therapy while biologic therapy could be interrupted. At present, conclusions about the influence of GC co-medication on the discontinuation outcome are not yet available. Future studies should include GCs in the experimental design and attempt to elucidate their role in inducing and maintaining biologic-free remission [43].

Why GCs Should Be Included in the Guidelines and Existing Gaps in the Knowledge

In accordance with the results presented, supported by evidence-based medicine and expert opinion, many rheumatologists advise that RA treatment should include GC co-medication. As recently suggested by the 2013 EULAR Task Force, low-dose oral GCs as a bridging add-on therapy on a DMARD background should be considered in the initial disease management. This regimen will allow rapid control of disease activity both in terms of clinical and subclinical reduction of the inflammatory process, thus ensuring long-standing structural benefits, which persist even after GC withdrawal. If the initial regimen is greater than 5 mg/day, dosage tapering to 5 mg should be attempted as early as is clinically feasible (possibly after 6 months of treatment). In the absence of available guidelines specifically addressing this issue, the decision to taper could be made along with clinician expertise and patient preferences. A possible role for GCs in maintaining clinical control after stopping other conventional and biologic DMARDs has not yet been fully elucidated, and there is limited information concerning GC withdrawal in the context of complex treatment regimens, including both biologic and nonbiologic DMARDs. The recently updated EULAR recommendations for the management of RA suggest that in case of persistent remission 'after having tapered GC, biologic DMARD tapering can be considered, especially if in combination with conventional DMARDs' [8]. This multistep-down strategy is confirmed in the Italian recommendations for the management of biologics for RA: GCs should be the first to be possibly reduced and discontinued; then, if a prolonged remission without GCs is obtained (over 12 months), a dose reduction in DMARDs and biotherapies may be considered [42]. Nonetheless, as stated above, little longitudinal evidence is available concerning the best strategy for down-titration/withdrawal of combination therapy once a patient has achieved a status of sustained response to combination treatment including GCs, conventional DMARDs and biologics, meaning that it is not yet possible to express clear recommendations [43]. Probably several disease-related factors, mainly disease duration, could influence the success of tapering strategies. For example, early RA patients could differ from established patients, who are likely to receive GCs chronically, with a possible subsequent and variable adrenocortical axis re-setting. Tapering must take into account possible adrenocorticoid function, sometimes with an ACTH stimulation test. It might also be possible that there is no absolute need to discontinue GCs at all when the dose becomes persistently below 5 mg/day. In more than 80% of RA patients seen in routine care at a single clinical setting, efficacy has been maintained with an indefinitely continued prednisone dosage of 3 mg/day with minimal side effects [17]. Thus, it would be optimal to compare in a randomized setting long-term results with lower versus higher prednisone dosages (such as 3 vs. 5–10 mg/day of prednisone), as well as no prednisone at all. Results from a single prednisone withdrawal clinical trial indicate that patients who were transferred from long-term prednisone doses of 1–4 mg/day to identical placebo tablets were significantly more likely to drop out due to perceived lack of efficacy over a subsequent 6- to 9-month period than those who were randomized to continue with 1 mg of prednisone daily: the long-term effectiveness and safety of long-term low-dose prednisone is encouraging [44]. It is unlikely that definitive data on GC withdrawal can come from randomized trials: some of the adverse events of GCs may require 5 years in many patients, whilst RCTs are generally of shorter duration. Many possible confounding variables cannot be kept under control in order to isolate prednisone dose as the only variable to analyze during withdrawal, and it is not possible to maintain randomization for long in a symptomatic condition such as RA. In addition, lack of standardization for the relevance of the side effects-to-benefit ratio for GC therapy can never be solved by randomized trials definitively: the significance of clinical and/or structural advantages may be considered differently by different individual patients and clinicians over the entity of concomitant side effects. In other words, the optimal tradeoff between risks and benefits due to GCs is not identical for all patients. Moreover, results in selected patients within RCTs might not be easily generalized and applied to actual individual patients: this could be problematic when considering the individual variation in response to GCs, for both clinical efficacy and safety issues, too. Considering all these

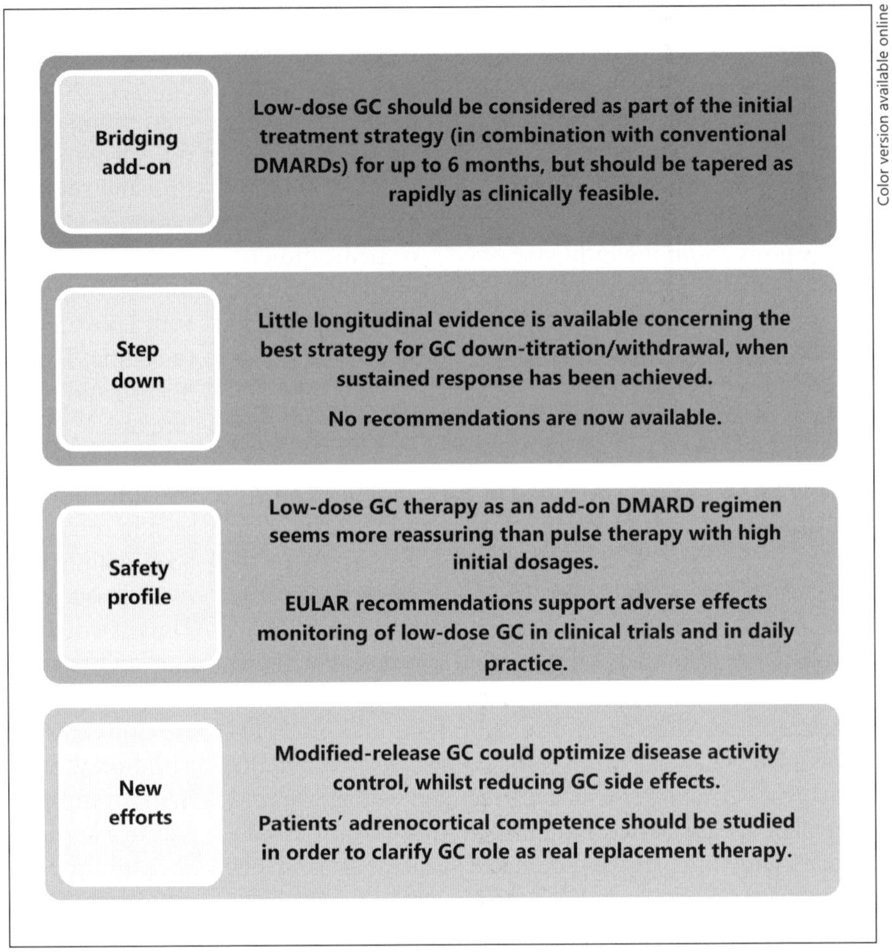

Fig. 1. Take home message: summary of current available achievements on GC therapy in RA patients.

limits, further complementary observational studies over long periods appear to be needed to advance knowledge toward optimal use of low-dose prednisone for patients with RA. Another gap to consider is that available recommendations did not specifically address the topic of the current availability of different GC formulations and routes of administration, or indications for intra-articular and intramuscular applications. New modified-release GC formulations optimize the timing of administration in order to coincide with the maximal inflammatory activity, so that therapeutic effect might be improved [45]. The circadian rhythm of pain, hormone levels and cytokine concentrations is a well-known phenomenon in patients with RA, and explains the circadian presentation of the most severe symptoms in the morning [46–48]. GC treatment traditionally has been given in the morning, when cytokines have already passed their peak. Recently, a modified-release tablet formulation has been developed that is released 4 h after ingestion. This allows patients to take the medication at 10 p.m. while drug delivery occurs at 2 a.m., with the capacity to suppress cytokines with optimal timing [49, 50]. The clinical efficacy of the modified-release prednisone in RA patients already taking traditional GCs has been assessed in CAPRA-1 and CAPRA-2 trials and in their open-label extensions [51–53]. In daily practice as well, as Cutolo et al. [54] recently demonstrated, real-life unselected patients experienced relevant short-term (4 months) benefits in disease activity signs and symptoms when switching from the ongoing traditional formulation (either oral prednisone or 6M-prednisolone) to the modified-release formulation. Long-term extension studies will also provide adjunctive information about structural effects.

GCs: Safety Profile

Although several positive effects of GCs have been demonstrated, their safety remains a matter of concern for both patients and clinicians. Most information comes from observational uncontrolled data in which doses, regimens, populations, disease and, therefore, results are highly heterogeneous, which prevents unequivocal conclusions. Clinical trials – which avoid the confounding by indication that inevitably affects observational studies, but carry relevant limitations regarding duration, inclusion criteria and standardization on the assessment of toxicity – do not provide comprehensive information, particularly concerning long-term toxicity. Furthermore, conclusions concerning toxicity, as previously stated, are not standardized; for example, is a slight risk of cataracts justified by joint preservation? Different patients and rheumatologists reach different shared decisions. The best available evidence suggests that low-dose GC therapy as an add-on to DMARD regimens appears acceptable, in contrast to high-dose oral GC or pulse therapy with high initial dosages [18, 55, 56]. The EULAR Task Force, through a dedicated literature search, developed recommendations aimed at monitoring the adverse effects of low-dose GC therapy (≤7.5 mg prednisone or equivalent daily) in clinical trials and daily practice, in order to specifically decide which potential adverse effects should be monitored, and how and how often this should be done. Since data concerning monitoring proved to be scarce and most articles were focused on the therapeutic rather than toxic effects of GCs, most recommendations were based on the consensus of experts [57]. Anyhow, as noted, continued very-low-dose GC might be a good compromise to assure clinical and structural efficacy while containing adverse events, and seems not to affect the hypothalamic-pituitary-adrenal axis significantly [17, 58].

Conclusions

GCs provide an effective and safe therapeutic option in low doses. As recently pointed out by the EULAR Task Force, low-dose oral GC should be included in any recommendation for the treatment of RA as an add-on therapy on a background of biologic or non-biologic DMARDs. This is especially true for early rather than established disease, with better long-term structural outcomes, even persisting after GC withdrawal. Such results could also rely on the deeper control of synovitis achieved through GC co-medication, as confirmed by ultrasound results. Low-dose GC schedules have a good safety profile as well, which brings them to use in the clinical practice, even if continuous and regular monitoring should be provided. Currently, the mandatory need remains to better clarify the tapering of GC medication and monitor it through specifically designed clinical trials and observational studies. New efforts have also been recently made to co-ordinate GC therapy with the chronobiological rhythms of cytokines involved in RA pathogenesis, with positive results of such modified-release agents, further emphasizing GCs as disease-modifying agents, with a replacement role in endogenous molecular pathways. These observations strongly support the central role of GCs in the management of RA patients, not differently from biologic and non-biologic DMARDs. For this reason, GCs should always be considered, when not contraindicated, for the treatment of RA (fig. 1).

References

1 Nam JL, Winthrop KL, van Vollenhoven RF, Pavelka K, Valesini G, Hensor EM, Worthy G, Landewé R, Smolen JS, Emery P, Buch MH: Current evidence for the management of rheumatoid arthritis with biological disease-modifying antirheumatic drugs: a systematic literature review informing the EULAR recommendations for the management of RA. Ann Rheum Dis 2010;69:976–986.

2 Knevel R, Schoels M, Huizinga TW, Aletaha D, Burmester GR, Combe B, Landewé RB, Smolen JS, Sokka T, van der Heijde DM: Current evidence for a strategic approach to the management of rheumatoid arthritis with disease-modifying antirheumatic drugs: a systematic literature review informing the EULAR recommendations for the management of rheumatoid arthritis. Ann Rheum Dis 2010;69:987–994.

3 Smolen JS, Landewé R, Breedveld FC, Dougados M, Emery P, Gaujoux-Viala C, Gorter S, Knevel R, Nam J, Schoels M, Aletaha D, Buch M, Gossec L, Huizinga T, Bijlsma JW, Burmester G, Combe B, Cutolo M, Gabay C, Gomez-Reino J, Kouloumas M, Kvien TK, Martin-Mola E, McInnes I, Pavelka K, van Riel P, Scholte M, Scott DL, Sokka T, Valesini G, van Vollenhoven R, Winthrop KL, Wong J, Zink A, van der Heijde D: EULAR recommendations for the management of rheumatoid arthritis with synthetic and biological disease-modifying antirheumatic drugs. Ann Rheum Dis 2010;69:964–975.

4 Aletaha D, Neogi T, Silman AJ, Funovits J, Felson DT, Bingham CO 3rd, Birnbaum NS, Burmester GR, Bykerk VP, Cohen MD, Combe B, Costenbader KH, Dougados M, Emery P, Ferraccioli G, Hazes JM, Hobbs K, Huizinga TW, Kavanaugh A, Kay J, Kvien TK, Laing T, Mease P, Ménard HA, Moreland LW, Naden RL, Pincus T, Smolen JS, Stanislawska-Biernat E, Symmons D, Tak PP, Upchurch KS, Vencovsky J, Wolfe F, Hawker G: 2010 rheumatoid arthritis classification criteria: an American College of Rheumatology/European League Against Rheumatism collaborative initiative. Ann Rheum Dis 2010;69:1580–1588.

5 Sakellariou G, Scirè CA, Zambon A, Caporali R, Montecucco C: Performance of the 2010 classification criteria for rheumatoid arthritis: a systematic literature review and a meta-analysis. PLoS One 2013;8:e56528.

6 Hoes JN, Jacobs JW, Boers M, Boumpas D, Buttgereit F, Caeyers N, Choy EH, Cutolo M, Da Silva JA, Esselens G, Guillevin L, Hafstrom I, Kirwan JR, Rovensky J, Russell A, Saag KG, Svensson B, Westhovens R, Zeidler H, Bijlsma JW: EULAR evidence-based recommendations on the management of systemic glucocorticoid therapy in rheumatic diseases. Ann Rheum Dis 2007;66:1560–1567.
7 Gorter SL, Bijlsma JW, Cutolo M, Gomez-Reino J, Kouloumas M, Smolen JS, Landewé R: Current evidence for the management of rheumatoid arthritis with glucocorticoids: a systematic literature review informing the EULAR recommendations for the management of rheumatoid arthritis. Ann Rheum Dis 2010;69:1010–1014.
8 Smolen JS, Landewé R, Breedveld FC, Buch M, Burmester G, Dougados M, Emery P, Gaujoux-Viala C, Gossec L, Nam J, Ramiro S, Winthrop K, de Wit M, Aletaha D, Betteridge N, Bijlsma JW, Boers M, Buttgereit F, Combe B, Cutolo M, Damjanov N, Hazes JM, Kouloumas M, Kvien TK, Mariette X, Pavelka K, van Riel PL, Rubbert-Roth A, Scholte-Voshaar M, Scott DL, Sokka-Isler T, Wong JB, van der Heijde D: EULAR recommendations for the management of rheumatoid arthritis with synthetic and biological disease-modifying antirheumatic drugs: 2013 update. Ann Rheum Dis 2014;73:492–509.
9 Smolen JS, Landewe R, Breedveld FC, Dougados M, Emery P, Gaujoux-Viala C, Gorter S, Knevel R, Nam J, Schoels M, Aletaha D, Buch M, Gossec L, Huizinga T, Bijlsma JW, Burmester G, Combe B, Cutolo M, Gabay C, Gomez-Reino J, Kouloumas M, Kvien TK, Martin-Mola E, McInnes I, Pavelka K, van Riel P, Scholte M, Scott DL, Sokka T, Valesini G, van Vollenhoven R, Winthrop KL, Wong J, Zink A, van der Heijde D: EULAR recommendations for the management of rheumatoid arthritis with synthetic and biological disease-modifying anti-rheumatic drugs. Ann Rheum Dis 2010;69:964–975.
10 Saag KG, Teng GG, Patkar NM, Anuntiyo J, Finney C, Curtis JR, Paulus HE, Mudano A, Pisu M, Elkins-Melton M, Outman R, Allison JJ, Suarez Almazor M, Bridges SL Jr, Chatham WW, Hochberg M, MacLean C, Mikuls T, Moreland LW, O'Dell J, Turkiewicz AM, Furst DE, American College of Rheumatology: American College of Rheumatology 2008 recommendations for the use of non-biologic and biologic disease-modifying antirheumatic drugs in rheumatoid arthritis. Arthritis Rheum 2008;59:762–784.
11 Singh JA, Furst DE, Bharat A, Curtis JR, Kavanaugh AF, Kremer JM, Moreland LW, O'Dell J, Winthrop KL, Beukelman T, Bridges SL Jr, Chatham WW, Paulus HE, Suarez-Almazor M, Bombardier C, Dougados M, Khanna D, King CM, Leong AL, Matteson EL, Schousboe JT, Moynihan E, Kolba KS, Jain A, Volkmann ER, Agrawal H, Bae S, Mudano AS, Patkar NM, Saag KG: 2012 update of the 2008 American College of Rheumatology recommendations for the use of disease-modifying antirheumatic drugs and biologic agents in the treatment of rheumatoid arthritis. Arthritis Care Res 2012;64:625–639.
12 National Collaborating Centre for Chronic Conditions (UK): Rheumatoid Arthritis: National Clinical Guideline for Management and Treatment in Adults. NICE Clinical Guidelines, No. 79. London, Royal College of Physicians, 2009.
13 Gaujoux-Viala C, Nam J, Ramiro S, Landewé R, Buch MH, Smolen JS, Gossec L: Efficacy of conventional synthetic disease-modifying anti-rheumatic drugs, glucocorticoids and tofacitinib: a systematic literature review informing the 2013 update of the EULAR recommendations for management of rheumatoid arthritis. Ann Rheum Dis 2014;73: 510–515.
14 van Everdingen AA, Jacobs JW, Siewertsz van Reesema DR, Bijlsma JW: Low-dose prednisone therapy for patients with early active rheumatoid arthritis: clinical efficacy, disease-modifying properties, and side effects: a randomized, double-blind, placebo-controlled clinical trial. Ann Intern Med 2002; 136:1–12.
15 Caporali R, Todoerti M, Sakellariou G, Montecucco C: Glucocorticoids in rheumatoid arthritis. Drugs 2013;73:31–43.
16 Da Silva JA, Jacobs JW, Kirwan JR, Boers M, Saag KG, Inês LB, de Koning EJ, Buttgereit F, Cutolo M, Capell H, Rau R, Bijlsma JW: Safety of low dose glucocorticoid treatment in rheumatoid arthritis: published evidence and prospective trial data. Ann Rheum Dis 2006; 65:285–293.
17 Pincus T, Sokka T, Castrejon I, Cutolo M: Decline of mean initial prednisone dosage from 10.3 to 3.6 mg/day to treat rheumatoid arthritis between 1980 and 2004 in one clinical setting, with long-term effectiveness of dosages less than 5 mg/day. Arthritis Care Res 2013; 65:729–736.
18 Pincus T, Sokka T, Kautiainen H: Patients seen for standard rheumatoid arthritis care have significantly better articular, radiographic, laboratory, and functional status in 2000 than in 1985. Arthritis Rheum 2005;52: 1009–1019.
19 Pincus T, Castrejón I, Sokka T: Long-term prednisone in doses of less than 5 mg/day for treatment of rheumatoid arthritis: personal experience over 25 years. Clin Exp Rheumatol 2011;29(5 suppl 68):S130–S138.
20 Landewe RB, Boers M, Verhoeven AC, Westhovens R, van de Laar MA, Markusse HM, van Denderen JC, Westedt ML, Peeters AJ, Dijkmans BA, Jacobs P, Boonen A, van der Heijde DM, van der Linden S: COBRA combination therapy in patients with early rheumatoid arthritis: long-term structural benefits of a brief intervention. Arthritis Rheum 2002;46:347–356.
21 Goekoop-Ruiterman YP, de Vries-Bouwstra JK, Allaart CF, van Zeben D, Kerstens PJ, Hazes JM, Zwinderman AH, Ronday HK, Han KH, Westedt ML, Gerards AH, van Groenendael JH, Lems WF, van Krugten MV, Breedveld FC, Dijkmans BA: Clinical and radiographic outcomes of four different treatment strategies in patients with early rheumatoid arthritis (the BeSt study): a randomized, controlled trial. Arthritis Rheum 2005;52: 3381–3390.
22 Graudal N, Jürgens G: Similar effects of disease-modifying antirheumatic drugs, glucocorticoids, and biologic agents on radiographic progression in rheumatoid arthritis: meta-analysis of 70 randomized placebo-controlled or drug-controlled studies, including 112 comparisons. Arthritis Rheum 2010;62: 2852–2863.
23 den Uyl D, Ter Wee M, Boers M, Kerstens P, Voskuyl A, Nurmohamed M, Raterman H, van Schaardenburg D, van Dillen N, Dijkmans B, Lems W: A non-inferiority trial of an attenuated combination strategy ('COBRA-light') compared to the original COBRA strategy: clinical results after 26 weeks. Ann Rheum Dis 2014;73:1071–1078.
24 Kirwan JR, The Arthritis and Rheumatism Council Low-Dose Glucocorticoid Study Group: The effect of glucocorticoids on joint destruction in rheumatoid arthritis. N Engl J Med 1995;333:142–146.
25 Svensson B, Boonen A, Albertsson K, van der Heijde D, Keller C, Hafström I: Low-dose prednisolone in addition to the initial disease-modifying antirheumatic drug in patients with early active rheumatoid arthritis reduces joint destruction and increases the remission rate: a two-year randomized trial. Arthritis Rheum 2005;52:3360–3370.
26 Wassenberg S, Rau R, Steinfeld P, Zeidler H: Very low-dose prednisolone in early rheumatoid arthritis retards radiographic progression over two years: a multicenter, double-blind, placebo-controlled trial. Arthritis Rheum 2005;52:3371–3380.
27 Todoerti M, Scire CA, Boffini N, Bugatti S, Montecucco C, Caporali R: Early disease control by low-dose prednisone comedication may affect the quality of remission in patients with early rheumatoid arthritis. Ann NY Acad Sci 2010;1193:139–145.

28 Capell HA, Madhok R, Hunter JA, Porter D, Morrison E, Larkin J, Thomson EA, Hampson R, Poon FW: Lack of radiological and clinical benefit over two years of low dose prednisolone for rheumatoid arthritis: results of a randomized controlled trial. Ann Rheum Dis 2004;63:797–803.
29 Hansen M, Podenphant J, Florescu A, Stoltenberg M, Borch A, Kluger E, Sørensen SF, Hansen TM: A randomised trial of differentiated prednisolone treatment in active rheumatoid arthritis: clinical benefits and skeletal side effects. Ann Rheum Dis 1999;58:713–718.
30 Bakker MF, Jacobs JW, Welsing PM, Verstappen SM, Tekstra J, Ton E, Geurts MA, van der Werf JH, van Albada-Kuipers GA, Jahangier-de Veen ZN, van der Veen MJ, Verhoef CM, Lafeber FP, Bijlsma JW, Utrecht Rheumatoid Arthritis Cohort Study Group: Low-dose prednisone inclusion in a methotrexate-based, tight control strategy for early rheumatoid arthritis: a randomized trial. Ann Intern Med 2012;156:329–339.
31 Brown AK, Quinn MA, Karim Z, Conaghan PG, Peterfy CG, Hensor E, Wakefield RJ, O'Connor PJ, Emery P: Presence of significant synovitis in rheumatoid arthritis patients with disease-modifying antirheumatic drug-induced clinical remission: evidence from an imaging study may explain structural progression. Arthritis Rheum 2006;54:3761–3773.
32 Filippucci E, Farina A, Carotti M, Salaffi F, Grassi W: Grey scale and power Doppler sonographic changes induced by intra-articular steroid injection treatment. Ann Rheum Dis 2004;63:740–743.
33 Scire CA, Montecucco C, Codullo V, Epis O, Todoerti M, Caporali R: Ultrasonographic evaluation of joint involvement in early rheumatoid arthritis in clinical remission: power Doppler signal predicts short-term relapse. Rheumatology 2009;48:1092–1097.
34 Montecucco C, Todoerti M, Sakellariou G, Scirè CA, Caporali R: Low-dose oral prednisone improves clinical and ultrasonographic remission rates in early rheumatoid arthritis: results of a 12-month open-label randomised study. Arthritis Res Ther 2012;14:R112.
35 Kirwan JR, Bijlsma JW, Boers M, Shea BJ: Effects of glucocorticoids on radiological progression in rheumatoid arthritis. Cochrane Database Syst Rev 2007:CD006356.
36 Jacobs JW, van Everdingen AA, Verstappen SM, Bijlsma JW: Follow-up radiographic data on patients with rheumatoid arthritis who participated in a two-year trial of prednisone therapy or placebo. Arthritis Rheum 2006;54:1422–1428.
37 Hafstrom I, Albertsson K, Boonen A, van der Heijde D, Landewé R, Svensson B, BARFOT Study Group: Remission achieved after 2 years treatment with low-dose prednisolone in addition to disease-modifying anti-rheumatic drugs in early rheumatoid arthritis is associated with reduced joint destruction still present after 4 years: an open 2-year continuation study. Ann Rheum Dis 2009;68:508–513.
38 Landewé RB, Boers M, Verhoeven AC, Westhovens R, van de Laar MA, Markusse HM, van Denderen JC, Westedt ML, Peeters AJ, Dijkmans BA, Jacobs P, Boonen A, van der Heijde DM, van der Linden S: COBRA combination therapy in patients with early rheumatoid arthritis: long-term structural benefits of a brief intervention. Arthritis Rheum 2002;46:347–356.
39 van Tuyl LHD, Boers M, Lems WF, Landewé RB, Han H, van der Linden S, van de Laar M, Westhovens R, van Denderen JC, Westedt ML, Peeters AJ, Jacobs P, Huizinga TW, van de Brink H, Dijkmans BA, Voskuyl AE: Survival, comorbidities and joint damage 11 years after the COBRA combination therapy trial in early rheumatoid arthritis. Ann Rheum Dis 2010;69:807–812.
40 Jacobs JWG: Lessons for the use of non-biologic anchor treatments for rheumatoid arthritis in the era of biologic therapies. Rheumatology 2012;51:iv27–iv33.
41 Volkmann ER, Rezai I S, Tarp S, Woodworth TG, Furst DE: We still don't know how to taper glucocorticoids in rheumatoid arthritis, and we can do better. J Rheumatol 2013;40;1646–1649.
42 Caporali R, Conti F, Alivernini S, Atzeni F, Seriolo B, Cutolo M, Valesini G, Ferraccioli G, Sarzi-Puttini P, Salvarani C, Guiducci S, Zampogna G, Gremese E, Pipitone N, Scrivo R, Bugatti S, Montecucco C, Matucci-Cerinic M, Italian Society for Rheumatology: Recommendations for the use of biologic therapy in rheumatoid arthritis: update from the Italian Society for Rheumatology. I. Efficacy. Clin Exp Rheumatol 2011;29:S7–S14.
43 Caporali R, Scirè CA, Todoerti M, Montecucco C: The role of low-dose glucocorticoids for rheumatoid arthritis in the biologic era. Clin Exp Rheumatol 2013;31(4 suppl 78):S9–S13.
44 Pincus T, Swearingen CJ, Luta G, Sokka T: Efficacy of prednisone 1–4 mg/day in patients with rheumatoid arthritis: a randomised, double-blind, placebo controlled withdrawal clinical trial Ann Rheum Dis 2009;68:1715–1720.
45 Cutolo M: Rheumatoid arthritis: circadian and circannual rhythms in RA. Nat Rev Rheumatol 2011;7:500–502.
46 Cutolo M, Villaggio B, Otsa K, Aakre O, Sulli A, Seriolo B: Altered circadian rhythms in rheumatoid arthritis patients play a role in the disease's symptoms. Autoimmun Rev 2005;4:497–502.
47 Cutolo M: Chronobiology and the treatment of rheumatoid arthritis. Curr Opin Rheumatol 2012;24:312–318.
48 Kirwan JR, Clarke L, Hunt LP, Perry MG, Straub RH, Jessop DS: Effect of novel therapeutic glucocorticoids on the circadian rhythms of hormones and cytokines in rheumatoid arthritis. Ann NY Acad Sci 2010;1193:127–133.
49 Spies CM, Cutolo M, Straub RH, Burmester GR, Buttgereit F: Prednisone chronotherapy. Clin Exp Rheumatol 2011;29(5 suppl 68):S42–S45.
50 Darendorf H, Ruebsamen K, Schaeffler A, Kirwan JR: Pharmacokinetics of modified release prednisone tablets are essentially unchanged from conventional immediate release prednisone tablets except from a programmed delay of 4–6 h. Ann Rheum Dis 2011;70(S3):604.
51 Buttgereit F, Doering G, Schaeffler A, Sierakowski S, Gromnica-Ihle E, Krueger K, Szechinski J, Alten R: Efficacy of modified-release versus standard prednisone to reduce duration of morning stiffness in the joints in rheumatoid arthritis (CAPRA-1): a double blind randomized controlled trial. Lancet 2008;371:205–214.
52 Buttgereit F, Doering G, Shaeffler A, Witte S, Sierakowski S, Gromnica-Ihle E, Jeka S, Krueger K, Szechinski J, Alten R: Targeting pathophysiological rhythms: prednisone chronotherapy shows sustainer efficacy in rheumatoid arthritis. Ann Rheum Dis 2010;69:1275–1280.
53 Buttgereit F, Mehta D, Kirwan J, Szechinski J, Boers M, Alten RE, Supronik J, Szombati I, Romer U, Witte S, Saag KG: Low-dose prednisone chronotherapy for rheumatoid arthritis: a randomised clinical trial (CAPRA-2). Ann Rheum Dis 2013;72:204–210.
54 Cutolo M, Iaccarino L, Doria A, Govoni M, Sulli A, Marcassa C: Efficacy of the switch to modified-release prednisone in rheumatoid arthritis patients treated with standard glucocorticoids. Clin Exp Rheumatol 2013;31:498–505.
55 Pincus T, Sokka T, Stein CM: Are long-term very low doses of prednisone for patients with rheumatoid arthritis as helpful as high doses are harmful? Ann Intern Med 2002;136:76–78.
56 Wei L, MacDonald TM, Walker BR: Taking glucocorticoids by prescription is associated with subsequent cardiovascular disease. Ann Intern Med 2004;141:764–770.
57 van der Goes MC, Jacobs JWJ, Boers M, Andrews T, Blom-Bakkers MA, Buttgereit F, Caeyers N, Cutolo M, Da Silva JA, Guillevin L, Kirwan JR, Rovensky J, Severijns G, Webber S, Westhovens R, Bijlsma JW: Monitoring adverse events of low-dose glucocorticoid therapy: EULAR recommendations for clinical trials and daily practice. Ann Rheum Dis 2010;69:1913–1919.
58 Larochelle G, Larochelle A, Ratner R, Borenstein D: Recovery of the hypothalamic-pituitary-adrenal (HPA) axis in patients with rheumatic diseases receiving low-dose prednisone. Am J Med 1993;95:258–264.

NeuroImmunoModulation

Neuroimmunomodulation 2015;22:112–118
DOI: 10.1159/000362732

Published online: September 12, 2014

Glucocorticoids in Juvenile Idiopathic Arthritis

Benedetta Schiappapietra[a] Giulia Varnier[a] Silvia Rosina[a]
Alessandro Consolaro[b] Alberto Martini[a, b] Angelo Ravelli[a, b]

[a]Università degli Studi di Genova, and [b]Istituto Giannina Gaslini, Genoa, Italy

Key Words
Juvenile idiopathic arthritis · Pediatric rheumatology · Glucocorticoids · Corticosteroids · Intra-articular injections

Abstract
Glucocorticoid (GC) drugs are a potent and rapidly effective therapeutic option for the treatment of juvenile idiopathic arthritis (JIA). These medications are mainly used for the management of the extra-articular features of systemic-onset disease. A course of low-dose prednisone may be considered for achieving a rapid disease control in patients with severe polyarthritis refractory to other therapies or while awaiting the full therapeutic effect of a recently initiated disease-modifying antirheumatic drug or biologic agent. Short-term systemic GC administration may also be indicated for chronic iridocyclitis unresponsive to topical therapy. The general objective of GC therapy is to limit the maximum dose and exposure to the highest doses to what is needed to achieve disease control, and then to gradually taper the dose until the minimum level sufficient to maintain disease quiescence over time is reached. High-dose intravenous 'pulse' methylprednisolone administration is sometimes chosen to treat the most severe or acute disease manifestations of systemic JIA, particularly macrophage activation syndrome. Intra-articular GC injection is a safe and rapidly effective treatment for synovitis in children with chronic arthritis. Triamcinolone hexacetonide is the optimal GC preparation for pediatric patients. Local injection therapy is used most frequently to treat oligoarthritis, but the strategy of performing multiple injections to induce disease remission, while simultaneously initiating therapy with second-line or biologic agents, has also been proposed for children with polyarticular JIA. Administration of GCs is associated with potentially deleterious adverse effects, some of which can be irreversible. This highlights the need of a judicious use of these medications and careful monitoring of their toxicity. The recently published recommendations for the management of JIA provide useful guidance to the clinicians for the administration of GCs in children with chronic arthritis.

Introduction

Glucocorticoid (GC) medications represent a potent and rapidly effective therapeutic option for the management of juvenile idiopathic arthritis (JIA) [1]. However, GCs are associated with substantial toxicity when administered systemically in high and even moderate doses. Some side effects may result in non-reversible damage, such as growth failure, which is especially worrisome in

KARGER

E-Mail karger@karger.com
www.karger.com/nim

1021–7401/14/0222–0112$39.50/0

Angelo Ravelli, MD
Pediatria II, Istituto G. Gaslini
Largo G. Gaslini 5
IT–16147 Genoa (Italy)
E-Mail angeloravelli@ospedale-gaslini.ge.it

young children. Therefore, when the use of these drugs is considered, the risk/benefit ratio must be carefully weighted.

The overall aim of GC therapy is to limit the maximum dose and the exposure to the highest doses that are needed to achieve disease control, and then to taper gradually the dose until the minimum level sufficient to maintain disease quiescence over time is reached. A child treated with these drugs should be under the care of a physician who is experienced in the management of the specific disease and in handling the risk of GC side effects.

Indications

In JIA, the use of systemic GCs is mainly restricted to the management of the extra-articular manifestations of systemic-onset disease. These include high fever unresponsive to non-steroidal anti-inflammatory drugs (NSAIDs), severe anemia, myocarditis or pericarditis, and macrophage activation syndrome (MAS) [2–5]. High-dose 'pulse' intravenous methylprednisolone (10–30 mg/kg/day to a maximum of 1 g/day on 1–3 consecutive days) is effective in controlling these features, but the effect is often short-lived. Therefore, continued GC therapy with oral prednisone (1–2 mg/kg/day to a maximum of 60 mg/day in single or divided daily doses) is frequently necessary. A short course of low-dose prednisone (e.g. 0.5 mg/kg/day) may be considered for alleviating pain and stiffness in patients with severe polyarthritis refractory to other therapies or while awaiting the full therapeutic effect of a recently initiated disease-modifying antirheumatic drug (DMARD) or biologic agent. Short-term systemic GC administration may also be indicated for chronic iridocyclitis unresponsive to topical therapy.

Adverse Effects

Overall, the side effects of GCs in children are similar to those observed in adults. However, some adverse events are unique to pediatric patients. The most serious long-term consequence of GC therapy in pediatric patients is growth suppression. It occurs in children who receive prolonged therapy in doses greater than 0.2–0.3 mg/kg/day of prednisone, increases with higher doses and is almost universally seen when divided doses are used [6]. However, wide inter-individual variation exists in the severity of growth suppression and the minimal dose required to suppress growth.

The mechanism of GC-induced growth suppression in children is unclear [7]. GCs have been shown to inhibit the production of somatomedin C (insulin-like growth factor I). In addition, their general inhibitory effects on cell growth and cell division probably contribute to growth failure. Growth suppression, however, although worsened by GC therapy, may also be a consequence of the underlying disease process. In JIA, particularly in the systemic-onset subtype, growth retardation can occur without GC therapy [8]. There is evidence suggesting that growth retardation is much more severe in children with JIA than in those with systemic lupus erythematosus receiving equivalent doses. The effect of growth hormones in improving height in children with GC-induced inhibition of growth is controversial.

Another potential harmful effect of continued GC administration in young children is delayed puberty, which is due to the long-lasting suppression of the hypothalamic-pituitary-adrenal (HPA) axis and is often associated with growth failure [9, 10]. Although pubertal delay is generally a temporary phenomenon, it can have irreversible consequences because it may contribute to hamper some important physiological milestones (that are also affected by GCs), such as growth spurt or bone mass accretion. These losses may not be regained once puberty develops and could lead to ultimate short stature and premature osteoporosis.

Minimizing Toxicity

The deleterious effects of GCs may be lessened by choosing a preparation with a relatively short half-life and the lowest dose that is efficacious. Prednisone is the drug most often selected for oral therapy. It has an optimal risk/benefit ratio, due to its enhanced GC and minimal mineralocorticoid actions. Some reports have claimed that deflazacort, an oxazoline derivative of prednisone, may have a bone-sparing effect compared with prednisone, although the evidence is unclear. Both the anti-inflammatory effect and the toxicity of GCs increase with larger doses and more frequent administration.

Morning administration has less capacity to suppress the pituitary than does administration later in the day (which blunts the surge of adrenocorticotropic hormone that normally occurs during sleep). The reduction of GC dose must be gradual and should be tailored to the child and the disease. At moderate-to-high doses (e.g. 40–60 mg/day) reductions of 5–10 mg are usually possible, whereas at lower doses (e.g. 5–10 mg/day) smaller reductions are generally needed. Further dose tapering should lead to a switch, whenever possible, to an alternate-day regimen. A too rapid dose decrease may cause noxious withdrawal effects, such as steroid pseudorheumatism or pseudotumor cerebri. There is no experience in children with JIA on the use of slow-release GC formulations [11].

There are no established guidelines for the prevention of GC-induced osteoporosis in pediatric patients. Several open studies have suggested that children with rheumatic diseases receiving GCs may benefit from calcium and vitamin D supplementation [1]. The bisphosphonates have also been studied as a potential treatment for GC-induced osteoporosis [12, 13]. However, many uncertainties persist regarding the use of these drugs in pediatrics, including which bisphosphonate is preferred, what the initial dose should be, and how long treatment should be continued. Furthermore, little is known about the duration of the anti-resorptive effect once bisphosphonates are discontinued in younger patients.

Prolonged GC therapy may lead to suppression of HPA function that can be slow in returning to normal. If not recognized, this complication places the child at risk for vascular collapse, adrenal crisis and death in situations that necessitate increased availability of cortisol. Under conditions of stress (serious infection, trauma, surgery), all children who are at risk for HPA axis suppression require supplemental GCs.

Intravenous Pulse GC Therapy

As noted above, high-dose 'pulse' intravenous GC therapy is sometimes used in the management of refractory systemic features of systemic-onset JIA or MAS. This approach aims to achieve an immediate, profound anti-inflammatory effect and to lessen toxicity associated with long-term continuous therapy in moderate to high daily doses. The drug of choice has been methylprednisolone, given in doses of 10–30 mg/kg per pulse up to a maximum of 1 g, administered according to a variety of protocols: a pulse each day for 3–5 days, alternate-day pulses for 3 doses, or a single administration repeated as clinical events warrant.

In the clinical setting, the calculated drug dose is usually added to 100 ml of 5% dextrose in water and infused over 1–3 h. Patient monitoring includes assessment of temperature, pulse rate, respiratory rate and blood pressure before beginning infusion. Pulse rate and blood pressure should then be checked every 15 min for the first hour and then every 30 min. Infusions should be slowed or discontinued if there are any significant changes in blood pressure or pulse rate.

The most commonly reported (10% of patients) short-term adverse effect of intravenous GC pulse therapy in children is abnormal behavior, with altered mood, hyperactivity, psychotic symptoms, disorientation and sleep disturbances. Other side effects include headache, abdominal discomfort, vomiting, hives, hypertension, dizziness, lethargy, hypotension, tachycardia and hyperglycemia. Little information is available about whether pulse therapy is associated with an increased risk for long-term side effects, such as osteoporosis or avascular necrosis of bone.

Intra-Articular GCs

Intra-articular GC injections are widely used in the management of children with JIA to induce rapid relief of inflammation symptoms and functional improvement, and to obviate the need for regular systemic therapy [14–16]. However, despite long use in pediatric rheumatology practice, much of the evidence supporting IAC therapy remains anecdotal or based on open, non-controlled studies. Furthermore, wide disparities likely exist in the indications for intra-articular GCs, injection technique, and protocols for sedation and post-injection management across different settings.

Although potentially effective on all subtypes of JIA, intra-articular GC injections are used most frequently to treat oligoarthritis. This therapy may prevent some important musculo-skeletal abnormalities in this JIA subset, such as flexion contractures, valgus deformity and leg-length discrepancy. Furthermore, intra-articular GC therapy has been proven to facilitate the discontinuation of oral GCs, resolve Baker's cysts and improve tenosynovitis [17].

The strategy of performing multiple intra-articular GC injections is used by some pediatric rheumatologists in children with polyarticular JIA to induce prompt remission of synovitis, while simultaneously initiating therapy with a DMARD and/or biologic agent. This approach is regarded as an alternative to systemic GCs to pursue a so-called 'bridge' effect, that is, to achieve a quick control of inflammatory symptoms while awaiting the full therapeutic effect of the systemic medication.

The duration of response to intra-articular GCs is dependent on the preparation used, with less soluble preparations providing a longer duration of response. Triamcinolone hexacetonide, the least soluble agent, is recog-

Table 1. Type and doses of GCs used for local injection therapy

Joint/site	Preparation	Dose		
		mg/kg	mg	Maximum, mg
Shoulder	TH	1		40
Elbow	TH	0.75		30
Wrist	TH	0.25–0.5[a]		20
Metacarpophalangeal and interphalangeal	MP		5–10[a]	
Hip	TH	1		40
Knee	TH	1		40
Ankle	TH	0.75		30
Subtalar and intertarsal	MP		20–40[a]	
Metatarsophalangeal and foot interphalangeal	MP		5–10[a]	
Tendon sheaths	MP		20–40[a]	

Adapted from Scott et al. [16]. TH = Triamcinolone hexacetonide; MP = methylprednisolone acetate. [a] Depending on child's size.

nized among pediatric rheumatologists as the medication of choice for intra-articular administration in JIA. The GC preparations and dosage regimen of intra-articular injections currently used in the authors' center is presented in table 1. In the post-injection period, the authors' recommendation is to avoid weight bearing for the first 24 h (72 h in case of injection in the hip) and to avoid high-impact physical activity in the 24–72 h after a joint injection. In case of relapse of synovitis, re-injection is commonly performed. Although there are no established guidelines for this practice, most rheumatologists will limit the frequency of re-injections to 3 times per year, with repeated procedures being performed at least 3 months apart.

The outcome and predictive variables of single and multiple intra-articular GC injections were investigated recently in 440 children with JIA [18]. The cumulative probability of remission of synovitis for patients injected in 1, 2 or 3 or more joints was 70, 45 and 44%, respectively, at 1 year; 61, 32 and 30%, respectively, at 2 years, and 37, 22 and 19%, respectively, at 3 years. Patients with systemic arthritis developed a synovitis flare more frequently and precociously than did patients with polyarthritis and oligoarthritis. The risk of synovitis flare was higher in patients who had positive C-reactive protein, negative anti-nuclear antibody and were injected in the ankle. The potential indications of multiple intra-articular GC injections (i.e. injections in 3 or more joints) in the various JIA categories were discussed in a subsequent report, based on the results obtained with this therapeutic procedure in 220 patients who had a total of 1,096 joints injected. The cumulative probability of survival without synovitis flare was 50.0, 31.5 and 19.5% at 1, 2 and 3 years, respectively. On Cox regression analysis, positive C-reactive protein value, negative anti-nuclear antibody, lack of concomitant methotrexate administration and a polyarticular (vs. an oligoarticular) disease course were the strongest predictors for synovitis flare [19].

The most common adverse effect of intra-articular GC injections is subcutaneous atrophic skin changes at the site of injection, particularly of small joints such as wrists and ankles in young children. It is caused by extravasation of the injected medication from the joint space. Subcutaneous atrophy resolves over time in most patients, but persists in some. The risk of this complication is minimized by following a careful injection technique, ensuring accuracy of needle placement in the joint space, and clearing the needle track with injection of saline or local anesthetic as the needle is withdrawn from the joint. No detrimental effect of intra-articular GCs on intra-articular cartilage or statural growth has been observed [20]. The potential role of GC injection in the hip in causing avascular necrosis of the femoral head is unclear. Reported studies suggest that the risk is small and is probably increased by the simultaneous administration of systemic GCs [21, 22].

Although systemic absorption of GCs has been found to cause significant adrenal suppression and transient clinical manifestations ranging from minor cosmetic changes to Cushingoid features, it is not associated with long-term adverse effects and is short-lived. Another known complication of intra-articular GC injections is the development of periarticular calcifications. The majority of these abnormalities are asymptomatic and are detected coincidentally on radiological follow-up.

A report of septic arthritis of the ankle 48 h after an intra-articular GC injection in the knee in a child with respiratory infection suggests that the procedure should be postponed if the child has signs of an ongoing infection [23]. A TB infection should be excluded before the intra-articular GC injection is made. Injected GCs may cause a crystal-induced synovitis, which may present with post-injection erythema and pain. This is thought to result from phagocytosis of GC crystals in the joint, leading to the release of inflammatory mediators [24]. These symptoms usually subside spontaneously or with local ice application within a few days.

Acute anaphylaxis following intra-articular GC administration has been described in adult patients, but has never been reported in children. Diabetic children may require a temporary increase in insulin doses.

Indications and Regimens of GC Therapy in Consensus Treatment Plans and Therapeutic Recommendations for JIA

In recent years, there have been several consensus initiatives aimed at providing guidance for the management of JIA through the formulation of consensus treatment plans or therapeutic recommendations. All these guidelines have included recommendations concerning intra-articular and systemic GCs.

By means of a modified Delphi method, consisting of an online questionnaire and a subsequent face-to-face consensus conference, an expert panel of pediatric rheumatologists developed algorithms for initiating, increasing or tapering GCs in systemic JIA [25]. Criteria for initiating or increasing GCs were the presence or development of anemia, myocarditis, pericarditis, pleuritis, peritonitis, and either complete or incomplete MAS. Criteria for tapering GCs included absence of fever for ≥3 days in the previous week, absence of poor physical functioning, and 7 laboratory criteria. A tapering schedule was also defined.

A consensus conference of members of the Childhood Arthritis and Rheumatology Research Alliance (CARRA) led to the development of 4 standardized treatment plans for new-onset systemic JIA [26]. The 4 therapeutic regimens included GCs only, or administration of methotrexate, anakinra or tocilizumab, with or without GCs. In all treatment plans, initial GC therapy was based on prednisone at 1 mg/kg (maximum 60 mg) daily and/or intravenous methylprednisolone pulses of 30 mg/kg (maximum 1 g) daily for 3 days.

Using the nominal group technique and Delphi method, the German Society for Pediatric Rheumatology created multidisciplinary, evidence- and consensus-based guidelines for the treatment of JIA [27]. Intra-articular GC injections were selected among the recommended therapeutic interventions and were indicated as a first-line treatment. Triamcinolone hexacetonide was deemed as more effective than triamcinolone acetonide in inducing local remission. Systemic GCs were recommended, owing to their fast action, in highly active JIA. More specifically, their use was advised for the treatment of systemic arthritis, rheumatoid factor-positive polyarthritis, potentially severe organ manifestations, such as uveitis or pericardial effusion, and as bridging therapy while awaiting the complete therapeutic effect of DMARDs. Long-term use of systemic GCs was discouraged.

The 2011 American College of Rheumatology (ACR) recommendations for the treatment of JIA were developed by an international panel of expert pediatric rheumatologists, following the Research and Development/University of California Los Angeles (RAND/UCLA) Appropriateness Method [28]. The panel recommended the use of GC joint injections for active arthritis, regardless of concurrent therapy with no DMARDs or non-biologic or biologic DMARDs, or JIA category. Triamcinolone hexacetonide was regarded as the preparation of choice. Re-injection was deemed appropriate in children with a history of arthritis in ≤4 joints in case the intervention resulted in clinical improvement of arthritis for at least 4 months. Systemic GC administration was recommended only for patients with systemic arthritis and active systemic features (and without active arthritis). In this subgroup, use of this treatment as initial therapy, with or without additional concurrent medications, was suggested for patients with active fever and MD global of ≥7. Initiation of systemic GCs following up to 2 weeks of NSAIDs was recommended for all patients with active fever.

Two years later, progress toward understanding of the pathophysiology of systemic JIA and the recent advance in its management led the ACR to update the recommendations for the medical therapy for JIA [29]. Recommendations were listed separately for 3 different disease phenotypes. For patients with active systemic features and varying degrees of synovitis, initial systemic GC monotherapy (administered by oral or intravenous route) was advised for a maximum of 2 weeks as a therapeutic option in the presence of an MD global <5 and an active joint count (AJC) >4, or in case the patient had an MD global ≥5, irrespective of the AJC. Continuing GCs as monotherapy for ≥1 month for patients with continued disease activity was considered inappropriate. Introduction of GC monotherapy was recommended as an option for patients with continued disease activity following failed treatment with NSAID monotherapy in the presence of an MD global <5 and an AJC >0, or in case the patient had an MD global ≥5, irrespective of the AJC. Both systemic and intra-articular GCs were recommended as adjunct therapy at any time. For the second phenotype of patients without active systemic features and with varying degrees of active synovitis, only intra-articular GC injections were recommended as an initial treatment option in the presence of an AJC ≤4. The utility of GC injection as the only therapeutic intervention in patients with an AJC >4 was considered uncertain. Administration of systemic GC monotherapy was recommended for the third group of patients with features concerning MAS. Continuing GC as the sole therapy for ≥2 weeks in

Table 2. Summary of 2011 and 2013 ACR recommendations for the use of intra-articular and systemic GCs in JIA

Treatment group	Therapeutic intervention	Recommendation
All	GC joint injection	For active arthritis, regardless of concurrent therapy
History of arthritis in ≤4 joints	GC joint injection	For all patients with active arthritis (with or without additional therapy), irrespective of disease activity level, prognostic features or joint contracture
	Repeated GC joint injection	For patients in whom the previous injection has resulted in clinical improvement of arthritis for ≥4 months
Systemic JIA with active systemic features and varying degrees of synovitis	Systemic GC monotherapy	As initial therapeutic option for a maximum period of 2 weeks for patients with an MD global <5 and an AJC >4, or an MD global ≥5, irrespective of the AJC
	Systemic GC monotherapy	Continuation for ≥1 month for patients with continued disease activity inappropriate
	Systemic GC monotherapy	For patients with continued disease activity, following failed treatment with NSAID monotherapy, if MD global <5 and AJC >0, or MD global ≥5, irrespective of the AJC
	Systemic GC monotherapy	As adjunct therapy at any time
	GC joint injection	As adjunct therapy at any time
Systemic JIA without active systemic features and varying degrees of synovitis	GC joint injection	As an initial therapeutic option for patients with an AJC ≤4 Uncertain as the only therapeutic option for patients with an AJC >4
Systemic JIA with features concerning for MAS	Systemic GC monotherapy	Recommended as a therapeutic option Continuing GC monotherapy for ≥2 weeks in patients with continued features concerning MAS inappropriate

GC = Glucocorticoid; JIA = juvenile idiopathic arthritis; AJC = active joint count; NSAID = nonsteroidal anti-inflammatory drug; MAS = macrophage activation syndrome.

patients with this phenotype was considered inappropriate. The 2011 and 2013 ACR recommendations for local and systemic administration of GCs in JIA are summarized in table 2.

Conclusion

GCs remain an important therapeutic option for children with JIA. Systemic administration of these medications is indicated mainly for the management of the extra-articular manifestations of systemic-onset disease, particularly high fever unresponsive to NSAIDs, severe anemia, myocarditis or pericarditis, and MAS. However, the use of systemic GCs in this condition will likely decrease in the future as a consequence of the marked effectiveness shown by the IL-1 and IL-6 inhibitors in recent clinical trials [30–32]. Intra-articular GC injection is a safe and rapidly effective treatment for synovitis in children with JIA and helps prevent joint contractures and other articular deformities. In addition, multiple GC injection therapy may represent a suitable strategy to induce quick and generalized remission of joint inflammation in children with polyarthritis, particularly in settings in which biologic medications are not available or affordable. Administration of GCs is associated with potentially deleterious adverse effects, some of which can be irreversible. This highlights the need for judicious use of these medications and careful monitoring of their side effects. The recently published recommendations for the treatment of JIA provide useful guidance to clinicians for the administration of GCs in children with JIA.

References

1 Ilowite NT, Laxer RM: Pharmacology and drug therapy; in Cassidy JT, Petty RE, Laxer RM, Lindley CB (eds): Textbook of Pediatric Rheumatology. 6th ed. Philadelphia, Elsevier Saunders, 2011, pp 71–126.
2 Ravelli A, Martini A: Juvenile idiopathic arthritis. Lancet 2007;369:767–778.

3 Hashkes PJ, Laxer RM: Medical treatment of juvenile idiopathic arthritis. JAMA 2005;294: 1671–1684.
4 Wallace CA: Current management of juvenile idiopathic arthritis. Best Pract Res Clin Rheumatol 2006;20:279–300.
5 Ravelli A, Martini A: Macrophage activation syndrome; in Lehman TH, Cimaz R (eds): Pediatric Rheumatology. Amsterdam, Elsevier 2008, pp 55–63.
6 Melo-Gomes JA: Problems related to systemic glucocorticoid therapy in children. J Rheumatol 1993;(Suppl. 37) 20:35–39.
7 Gedalia A, Shetty AK: Chronic steroid and immunosuppressant therapy in children. Pediatr Rev 2004;25:425–434.
8 De Benedetti F, Martini A: Is systemic juvenile rheumatoid arthritis an interleukin 6 mediated disease? J Rheumatol 1998;25:203–207.
9 Gutierrez-Suarez R, Ruperto N, Gastaldi R et al: A proposal for a pediatric version of the Systemic Lupus International Collaborating Clinics/American College of Rheumatology Damage Index based on the analysis of 1015 patients with juvenile-onset systemic lupus erythematosus. Arthritis Rheum 2006;54: 2989–2996.
10 Hiraki LT, Hamilton J, Silverman ED: Measuring permanent damage in pediatric systemic lupus erythematosus. Lupus 2007;16: 657–662.
11 Spies CM, Bijlsma JW, Burmester GR, Buttgereit F: Pharmacology of glucocorticoids in rheumatoid arthritis. Curr Opin Pharmacol 2010;10:302–307.
12 Bianchi ML, Cimaz R, Bardare M, et al: Efficacy and safety of alendronate for the treatment of osteoporosis in diffuse connective tissue diseases in children: a prospective multicenter study. Arthritis Rheum 2000;43: 1960–1966.
13 Marini JC: Do bisphosphonates make children's bones better or brittle? N Engl J Med 2003;349:423–426.
14 Dent PB, Walker N: Intra-articular corticosteroids in the treatment of juvenile rheumatoid arthritis. Curr Opin Rheumatol 1998;10: 475–480.
15 Cleary AG, Murphy HD, Davidson JE: Intra-articular corticosteroid injections in juvenile idiopathic arthritis. Arch Dis Child 2003;88: 192–196.
16 Scott C, Meiorin S, Filocamo G, et al: A reappraisal of intra-articular corticosteroid therapy in juvenile idiopathic arthritis. Clin Exp Rheumatol 2010;28:774–781.
17 Padeh S, Passwell JH: Intraarticular corticosteroid injection in the management of children with chronic arthritis. Arthritis Rheum 1998;41:1210–1214.
18 Lanni S, Bertamino M, Consolaro A, et al: Outcome and predicting factors of single and multiple intra-articular corticosteroid injections in children with juvenile idiopathic arthritis. Rheumatology 2011;50:1627–1634.
19 Huppertz HI, Tschammler A, Horwitz AE, Schwab KO: Intraarticular corticosteroids for chronic arthritis in children: efficacy and effects on cartilage and growth. J Pediatr 1995; 127:317–321.
20 Papadopoulou C, Kostik M, Gonzalez-Fernandez MI, et al: Delineating the role of multiple intraarticular corticosteroid injections in the management of juvenile idiopathic arthritis in the biologic era. Arthritis Care Res (Hoboken) 2013;65:1112–1120.
21 Neidel J, Boehnke M, Kuster RM: The efficacy and safety of intraarticular corticosteroid therapy for coxitis in juvenile rheumatoid arthritis. Arthritis Rheum 2002;46:1620–1628.
22 Tynjala P, Honkanen V, Lahdenne P: Intra-articular steroids in radiologically confirmed tarsal and hip synovitis of juvenile idiopathic arthritis. Clin Exp Rheumatol 2004;22:643–648.
23 Shore A, Rush PJ: Possible danger of intraarticular steroid injection in children with respiratory tract infections. Br J Rheumatol 1987;26:73.
24 Hertzberger-ten Cate R, de Vries-van der Vlugt BC, van Suijlekom-Smit LW, Cats A: Intra-articular steroids in pauciarticular juvenile chronic arthritis, type 1. Eur J Pediatr 1991;150:170–172.
25 Ilowite NT, Sandborg CI, Feldman BM, et al: Algorithm development for corticosteroid management in systemic juvenile idiopathic arthritis trial using consensus methodology. Pediatr Rheumatol Online J 2012;10:31.
26 Dewitt EM, Kimura Y, Beukelman T, et al: Consensus treatment plans for new-onset systemic juvenile idiopathic arthritis. Arthritis Care Res (Hoboken) 2012;64:1001–1010.
27 Dueckers G, Guellac N, Arbogast M, et al: Evidence and consensus based GKJR guidelines for the treatment of juvenile idiopathic arthritis. Clin Immunol 2012;142:176–193.
28 Beukelman T, Patkar NM, Saag KG, et al: 2011 American College of Rheumatology recommendations for the treatment of juvenile idiopathic arthritis: initiation and safety monitoring of therapeutic agents for the treatment of arthritis and systemic features. Arthritis Care Res (Hoboken) 2011;63:465–482.
29 Ringold S, Weiss PF, Beukelman T, et al: 2013 update of the 2011 American College of Rheumatology recommendations for the treatment of juvenile idiopathic arthritis: recommendations for the medical therapy of children with systemic juvenile idiopathic arthritis and tuberculosis screening among children receiving biologic medications. Arthritis Rheum 2013;65:2499–2512.
30 Yokota S, Imagawa T, Mori M, et al: Efficacy and safety of tocilizumab in patients with systemic-onset juvenile idiopathic arthritis: a randomised, double-blind, placebo-controlled, withdrawal phase III trial. Lancet 2008;371:998–1006.
31 De Benedetti F, Brunner HI, Ruperto N, et al: Randomized trial of tocilizumab in systemic juvenile idiopathic arthritis. N Engl J Med 2012;367:2385–2395.
32 Ruperto N, Brunner HI, Quartier P, et al: Two randomized trials of canakinumab in systemic juvenile idiopathic arthritis. N Engl J Med 2012;367:2396–2406.

NeuroImmunoModulation

Author Index Vol. 22, No. 1–2, 2015

E-Mail karger@karger.com
www.karger.com/nim

NeuroImmunoModulation

Subject Index Vol. 22, No. 1–2, 2015

KARGER

E-Mail karger@karger.com
www.karger.com/nim